DIARY OF AN ADORABLE FAT GIRL

THE FIRST TWO WEIGHT LOSS BOOKS

BERNICE BLOOM

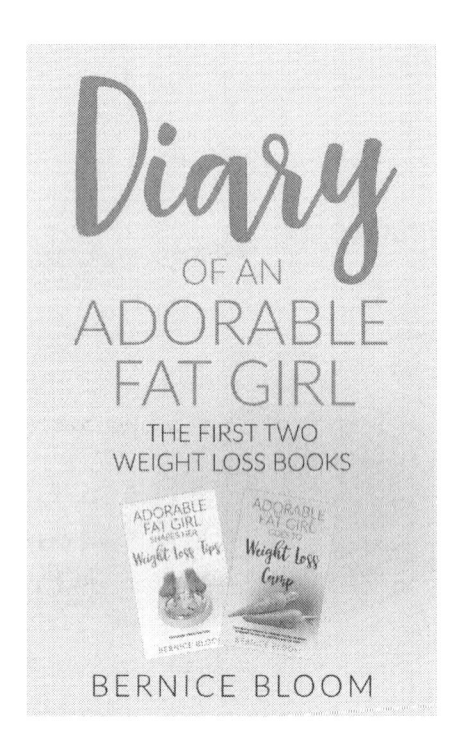

Published internationally by Gold Medals Media Ltd:

© Bernice Bloom 2019

Terms and Conditions:

The purchaser of this book is subject to the condition that he/she shall in no way resell it, nor any part of it, nor make copies of it to distribute freely.

❀ Created with Vellum

HELLO, WELCOME TO MY WORLD...

Hello,

Thanks so much for downloading this box-set of two Adorable Fat Girl books staring Mary Brown. I hope you enjoy them.

The books tell the story of Mary Brown and her bonkers weight-loss adventures. The first book details her weight loss tips and the second one is the story of when she went on a weight loss camp...

The books have sold almost 100,000 copies since they first went on sale. I'm so pleased there's a new, romantic heroine out there who is funny, gorgeous and NOT SKINNY!

Thank you for supporting her!

There are loads more books in the series...more mini books are being released all the time. There's even talk of a film: so, watch this space!

Thanks again for your support,

Bernie xx

INTRODUCTION

TO WEIGHT LOSS TIPS

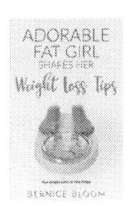

Dear readers,

Hello, my name's Bernice Bloom. It's presently quarter past six on a soft summer's evening and I'm lying on the floor doing leg lifts while I catch up with *Made In Chelsea*. And if that little nugget of information hasn't left you reeling in your seat then you don't know me very well.

Me - exercising in my own home? Squeezing in a little bit of gentle exercise while I relax over skinny, posh people in the evening? Incorporating exercise into my everyday life...exactly like they tell you to in every article about fitness ever written.

Me - doing something right? Yes - I know - I don't understand what's happened to me either.

But - somehow - despite years of failing to lose more than three pounds before putting eight pounds instantly back on again, this time I have got myself sorted and I've managed to properly lose weight. I feel amazing...not thin - not by a long way, I've lost half the weight I need to lose so there's still a way to go, but I've lost a lot, and losing weight is definitely an incentive to lose more weight because every pound you lose gives you confidence that you can lose more, so I'm full of hope that I'll lose the rest of it and soon be deliciously slim and *probably* giving Kate Moss a run for her money.

If you've read the novels about my character Mary Brown's exploits, you'll know that she joined a Fat Club and it transformed her life. Not only did she meet a whole load of thoroughly lovely people who she went on a lot of crazy adventures with, she also bagged herself a delicious new boyfriend and - crucially - she managed to shift the piles of lard that had settled on her stomach, thighs and hips.

She did it by following the five steps that they taught her at Fat Club and I'm going to explain them to you now. Everyone at Fat Club lost weight and you can too.

If you follow these steps you will lose weight - I promise!!!

Bernie x

www.bernicebloom.com

Introduction from Mary Brown, star of the Adorable Fat Girl series:

Before I lost weight, I used to wonder how people did it. I mean **really** wonder... I would see someone in the paper who'd lost two stone, or bump into an old friend who I hadn't seen for ages, and discover they had lost weight, toned up and were looking fantastic. And I'd think – how have you done it? HOW ON GOD'S FREAKING EARTH HAVE YOU DONE IT?

And the fascinating thing is, when I thought 'how have you done it?' I didn't mean it literally because I knew exactly what they'd done – they'd eaten less and exercised more. We all know what to do to lose weight. You know how the body works and I know how the body works. I know that if you put in less than you take out, you'll lose the weight. Simple! But – no, no, no – because the maddening truth is that it's very hard to do...not simple at all.

So when I saw someone who had lost weight, what I asked myself was – how did you mentally convince yourself to do what millions of us want to do?

What I wanted from them was a tip, a clue as to how they did it. I was dying for one magical little secret that would help me. I really didn't need them to say 'Eat broccoli, not a chocolate bar.' I didn't need to hear that they got off the bus a few stops early and walked up the stairs.'

I KNOW ALL THAT. TELL ME WHERE THE MAGIC KEY IS THAT WILL UNLOCK, IN MYSELF, THE ABILITY NOT TO EAT ALL THE TIME.

In the search for the magic key I went to Overeaters Anonymous and there I discovered the five tips for losing weight that have transformed my life. I'm going to tell you right off the bat what they are, then in this little book, I'll go through them in much more detail, and explain what it all means, with examples of how the people I met on Fat Club and various readers who have written in to me, got them to work. Then all you have to do is follow them and lose tonnes of weight, then next time your friend sees you she'll scream HOW HAVE YOU DONE IT? And you'll be able to smile and say 'yeah...it's all because of Bernice Bloom,' and I'll be famous and be invited to garden parties at Buckingham Palace. Everyone's a winner.

OK. So, the five tips are:

- Understand what your body wants
- Psych yourself in instead of psyching yourself out
- Be nice to yourself; treat yourself with respect
- WAW! Water and walking
- Making it a habit

Nice and straightforward? Not yet, but it will be. I promise, promise, promise it will be.

One of the things that going to Fat Club gave me was a confidence in my ability to lose weight. When everyone is positive around you, it's amazing how that rubs off and you feel positive too. I stopped beating myself up and started accepting that I wasn't overweight because I was greedy, lazy, slovenly or useless. I was overweight because I used food to make myself feel better, feel less bored, less lonely or less vulnerable.

The key thing that I did when I realised that was to break the emotional connection between food and feeling good. I started thinking of food as being exactly what it really was, instead of what it represented to me. Then I could start transforming myself into the person I wanted to be. Food is just there to stop you being hungry; that's all.

Keep saying that to yourself...that's all it is. FOOD IS JUST TO STOP HUNGER.

Say it, say it again. SHOUT IT.

You can lose weight if you only use food to combat hunger. Deep down you know you can do it. Face it, you can do anything if you really want to.

I mean, people have done extraordinary things in the world. People do crazily complicated wild and wonderful things every day. I've seen the news - blokes air ballooning round the world, swimming the channel and women giving birth to quadruplets on top of a mountain and things like that. Running marathons? How do people do that? I'm the same species as all these people yet I can't run further than the kitchen without needing open heart surgery and a lung transplant.

We both know that we CAN do it. But we don't, and that's mainly because we use food to try and change our emotional outlook, not just our physical hunger and learned behaviour.

I knew that I really must be able to change my outlook on the world, and get out of the bad habits I'd got into...stop eating the leftovers purely out of habit. Stop clearing everything on my plate because that's what I'd always been told to do as a child. I wasn't a child - I was a 20-stone woman. I had to learn a new approach to food.

What I learned more than anything from Fat Club was that people become overweight for lots of different reasons - eat too much ice cream, drink too much, too much chocolate...but the thing people have in common is that they are overweight because food has become more than nutrition to them.

If that's you, please read on...perhaps you've eaten when you're lonely, or bored, or you eat because the children are playing you up, eat because your boss is a pain. You might be eating to fill a little hole inside you that sits there because you don't feel loved or happy or worthy. You know that food doesn't help you but you eat it anyway because it's a quick and easy way to feel instantly full, protected and satisfied.

This is not a diet book – heavens, there are a million diet books out there – the world doesn't need any more. This is a book that should motivate you, comfort you and help you.

I happen to think it's a very important book because it will make you feel much, much better about yourself while you're losing weight and I happen to think that feeling good about yourself is the most important thing in the world, and certainly the thing that will help with weight loss.

Food is many people's way of reaching out, psychologically, for something to make them feel warm and happy and loved. Tell me - how the hell is a diet book that tells you to eat spinach leaves instead of chips going to help you feel warm and loved? It's not about understanding what to eat – WE ALL KNOW THAT - it's about understanding how to feel nice without reaching for cake. It's about breaking the habit.

If you are overweight it's not because you're a bad person, you didn't kill anyone, you didn't steal anything, or hit anyone, or do anything criminal. You just ate too much because you felt low, or got into a habit of eating while bored. That's not a crime. Most importantly, it can be changed. Reading this book is a great start because it will show you examples of lots and lots of people from my Fat Club and from readers who changed, and explain how they did it.

I really hope it helps you, I know it will make you feel better about yourself, and make you realise that 90% of the battle is about loving yourself a bit more and not feeling the need to medicate with food, silence the pain with food, or kill time with food. And it's simpler than you think…lots of people have written in to me and told me that they did it, and their stories are in this book.

This book is divided into five sections based on the five tips outlined earlier. At the beginning of each section is an explanation of the way in which that tip helped me, then stories from other people who have written in to me to explain how they lost weight.

I really hope you enjoy the book and if you want to read any of the funny novels about my life, they are all on:

www.bernicebloom.com

Or here on Amazon:

https://www.amazon.co.uk/Bernice-Bloom/e/B01MPZ5SBA/ref=sr_ntt_srch_lnk_1?qid=1544794288&sr=1-1

SECTION ONE

UNDERSTAND WHAT YOUR BODY NEEDS

WILD ANIMALS

OK. This is where the fun starts...your first step to a whole new body. I want to begin by telling you about my trip to a safari last year. (see Adorable Fat Girl on Safari: http://amzn.to/2fbEZ73)

When I was out in the wilds, watching the animals, the thing that struck me most of all was how none of them were fat. NONE of them. Not one single animal. If you sit in any cafe in town and people watch, you'll see all range of sizes pass by; certainly you won't have to sit there for very long before seeing someone who is overweight Why is that? What are animals going that we are not?

Happily, on safari, there was a rather handsome ranger on hand to explain:

The main reason that animals aren't overweight is because they don't eat more than they need. They eat to live. If an animal has just made a kill, he eats that animal, then goes out to make another kill when he's hungry. The relationship between animals and food is that they eat because food is the fuel to keep them going. They don't eat because the alpha lion has gone off with a young female, because they're bored or because they feel depressed. They eat when they are hungry.

How do they know when they are hungry? The same way as we

do: hunger pains. Hunger pains are your best friend! Learn to love them and cherish them.

Those pains or rumbles we feel are designed to tell us that sometime soon it would be good to have some food. They are a sign that you are ready to eat. Honestly - I know this sounds ridiculous - but those rumbles and pains are really important.

Conditioning has taught us that when our stomachs rumble it's a bad thing, and that we shouldn't let ourselves get so hungry that they rumble. Yes we should! The truth is that those hunger pains are a good thing. They indicate that your stomach wants food soon. They are a warning that you're getting low on fuel (it's like the fuel gauge on the car moving down - you're not about to stop through lack of petrol, but it would be good to put some petrol in the car in the not-too-distant future).

Treating food as fuel and eating when you feel hungry are the keys to survival in the wild. Could they be the key to weight loss too?

Over the next couple of weeks, try only to eat when you're hungry and at least once a week, make sure your stomach rumbles before you eat. Just try it. Give yourself a loud cheer every time you hear your stomach rumble...it's a good thing - welcome it and celebrate it.

The third point I want to make in this section contains what you should eat. What is your body asking for when you feel hungry and get those hunger pains? Fuel. Exactly like when a car asks for fuel. You can't just shove crisps, pizza and chocolate into a car engine or you'll run into problems, and you can't just shove crisps, chocolate and pizza into your mouth either, without there being problems.

Try hard to remember this: when you feel hunger pains your body wants nutrients. If you eat a big fruit salad, you may not feel the same satisfaction as if you eat great big fried breakfast, but you will give your body the nutrients it wants so you won't get as hungry later. You could eat a whole loaf of bread and it would fill you up, but your body won't feel satisfied because it won't have had the nutrients that it needs, so the hungry feelings will emanate again, as your body asks for nutrients again. If you eat rubbish again, the body will say it's hungry again an hour later, as it realises it doesn't have the nutrients it needs in the food you've supplied. So, you'll eat more and more and get fatter and fatter and always be hungry. Does that sound like you? It sounds a lot like I used to be. And it's a horrible way to live; always stuffing yourself full of food, and always feeling hungry and unsatisfied. Stop it now!

So - just to summarise - three things to remember:

- Think of the safari animals and try to think of food as fuel. Just eat to fuel yourself when you get hungry and pick the best fuel.
- Try to wait for hunger pains or at least murmurings of hunger before you eat. Treat hunger pains as real triumphs.
- Remember what the pains mean - they mean that your body needs nutrients...not just any old food - you won't be satisfied if you eat any old food, eat the most natural, unprocessed, healthy food you can, then the hunger pains will dissipate, the weight will fall off, you'll feel better and healthier and won't be drawn to unhealthy eating in the future.

I found the key to losing weight was to think about what my body needed, not what my mind or my emotions required. My body needed nutrients so that's what I gave it. As much food as I wanted, as long as everything I ate was doing me some good.

Here are some stories that readers have shared about their weight loss journeys and their keys to success with food control. I hope you enjoy their stories...

Sarah's story:
　　Hi, my name is Sarah. I'm 52-years-old and I have lost 54lbs. I went from 196lbs to 142lbs. I did it by not being a dustbin!

I'd tried to lose weight loads of times before, but would lose some weight, then get fed up, stop, and put it all back on again. Then, I did it. I lost the weight and kept it off because of one simple saying that has really worked for me - don't be a dustbin. It's quite simple, but that's the rule I have…and it's worked. I write DBAD on my hand every morning, and am conscious of it all the time. I urge you to try it – just implant that saying into your mind.

My story:

I realised I had a problem around food when someone saw me finishing the leftovers from a Chinese takeaway we'd had, and said "how can you still be hungry?"

The question took me by surprise - of course I wasn't hungry - we just had a huge meal, but I carried on eating just because it was there. I'd got it into my head that it was better if I ate the leftovers than threw them away. A mixture of not wanting to waste food that was there, and habit. It seemed daft to leave a couple of spring rolls and some spoonfuls of seaweed behind – so I just put them into my mouth despite not being at all hungry.

My friend said "the leftovers belong in the dustbin", and it suddenly struck me that I was treating myself a bit like a dustbin. Why was I shoving bits of food I didn't want into my mouth? Habit.

If there were any bits of bread lying around, or if there was a piece of pizza left -- I would eat it. I wasn't hungry, lonely, sad or any of the other things that drive you to eat. It was just habit that I'd shove any leftovers into my mouth. The kids would leave their crusts – I'd eat them. I'd serve up dinner and there'd be a little left in the pot – I'd eat it. Gradually, I'd put on a hell of a lot of weight.

So, I decided to stop. I created my DBAD label and set about trying hard to break the habits of a lifetime. It was much easier than I thought it would be. I think what happens when you start thinking to yourself "I will not be a dustbin" is it you think more carefully about everything you're putting into your mouth. Will this do me any good, or am I eating it because it's there? Why am I eating it? It forces you to take that two minute break before shoving something into your mouth that forces you to think about whether you really need it or want it.

Try it. As you're making dinner, don't shove bits of food into your mouth while you're cooking – have more respect for yourself. You're not a dustbin.

I've found that my habit of just eating any leftovers or anything left on the side disappeared when I refused to treat myself like a dustbin anymore. It also made me think about the whole concept of having "leftovers", and food lying around that could easily tempt me. I've got three teenage children, so I do a big supermarket shop every week, but what I've tried to do is be really specific about what to buy in the weekly shop -- what do I plan to cook for the meals that week? What do I need to buy?

Rather than wandering around and grabbing things off the shelves and throwing them into my basket, I think about the meals we are going to eat. I think DBAD as I'm walking down the aisles. Shopping properly means eating properly - it means there's less food being wasted, and less chance of me hoovering it up.

This in itself has definitely made a difference to the amount I'm eating, but I think it's more the fact that I am a subconsciously thinking before I eat that is making a real difference.

The gradual process of making yourself look at food differently means thinking about what's best for you. I started to think of fruit and veg as being treats, because they make me feel better and look great and so are the opposite of being a dustbin. Shoving bits of old pizza left in the box into my mouth, and the remains of a Chinese takeaway was never going to make me feel better – that stuff belongs in the bin, not in me.

If you shove pieces of cake in your mouth to make you feel better for five minutes, the impact of it can be colossal -- you stop caring, you don't value yourself. You start using food to make yourself feel better. I'd never have been able to do it by thinking about it logically – I did it by having a strict rule – don't be a dustbin, and the rest came naturally.

Just think about it... of all the things in the world you might want to be -- why would anyone want to be a dustbin? Every time you feel yourself behaving in a dustbin like fashion -- stop it. Become aware of any dustbin like tendencies.

There is no one reading this book who wants to be a dustbin, so stop it!

As I said, I wrote DBAD on my hand to remind myself "don't be a dustbin" -- it started to apply to everything I put into my mouth. Was I eating this because it was good for me, or was I just being a dustbin? I found this tactic really worked. This is a simple thing, but sometimes it's the simple things that people say that click something in your mind and make you behave differently.

The other thing about this small saying is that it's not setting you off on a tightly calorie controlled diet, or making you run six miles a day. It's just subtly getting you to alter your behavior around food. If someone has got a handful of chips left on their plates - don't eat them, you are not a dustbin. You are worth more than that. Much more than that.

Pippa's story:
Four golden rules

Hi, my name is Pippa. I'm 58-years-old and I have lost 43lbs. I went from 183lbs to 140lbs. I did it by being incredibly strict with myself and following these four golden rules.

My story:

I'm not the sort of person who normally follows rules ... if I'm making a cake, I find it really hard to follow the recipe, I like to throw things in a mixer and see what it tastes like. But somehow, perhaps because my mind is so chaotic and in need of order, I found that when I set myself very clear rules to follow, I was able to lose weight. I call these my four golden rules, and I took to wearing four gold-coloured bangles to remind myself constantly of these four rules. I think that if you are going to follow strict rules, you need to remember them all the time, and it was a constant reminder to me, every time I reached out to food, and saw the four bangles jangling on my wrist.

So, my four rules… these are my tips to you; if you follow them you will lose weight. Let me repeat that: YOU WILL LOSE WEIGHT. Now if you decide not to follow them, or that all sounds like too much like hard work, that's your decision but I'm telling you that these rules work. As I've already said, if you're the sort of person who thinks they might forget, a good way is with the four bracelet or four bangles approach.

My first golden rule was - when I was hungry I allowed myself to eat. But I could only eat when I was hungry; I didn't allow myself to eat until I was hungry. This helped teach me when I should be eating. If other people were eating and I wasn't hungry, I'd stop myself. I'd looked down at my bangles, and remind myself that I could only eat when I was hungry … when I could feel that hunger building up in my stomach.

The second rule, which goes hand in hand with this rule, was that I had to stop eating when I wasn't hungry anymore. I ignored all the rules from childhood, that you have to finish everything on your plate, and just ate until I wasn't hungry anymore. Remember, if you get hungry again, you can have more food. There's no shortage of food. This took a bit of getting used to, and I realised that most of the time when I'd eaten less than half of the food on my plate I wasn't hungry anymore, I was fine, but I was eating it because it was there. If you can stop yourself (look at the bangles) make yourself put your knife and fork down when you are no longer hungry, you'll find it makes a huge difference to the amount you consume. I think, looking back, that most of the food I was eating wasn't because I was hungry, but because it was there.

So, they are the two main golden rules. If you can follow them, you'll lose weight.

The other two rules I had were in order to make those to work.

So, rule number three was that I should eat whatever my body felt it needed. I was sure that my body would direct me to what it needed if I stopped just guzzling whatever was in front of me. I'd realised this when I was pregnant with my first child, and got mad urges for certain sorts of food as my body tried to feed the two of us. If the body was capable of doing that when I was pregnant, then clearly it was capable of doing it once I'd had the baby. I might just have to listen a bit more carefully for the cues. Now, if I am really hungry, and really fancy carbohydrates, I won't stop myself. If I'm hungry, I eat, but I try to eat what I feel my body wants me to eat, and – of course – I stop when I'm full.

My final rule, the final gold bangle on my wrist, is probably the nicest, but it's also very important - that rule is that I should really enjoy the food I was eating. So if I had a plate of food, I should relish all the different tastes and really enjoy it while I was eating it, rather than shovelling it down and feeling guilty about it as I had before. But then stop when I wasn't hungry anymore.

I made myself eat properly at a table and not while distracted at my desk, on the train, or while walking down the street. If you eat while you're reading a book or flicking through a newspaper, you're distracted from the process of eating, and you never know when you're full. Jangle those bangles, lay out a proper table, sit down and enjoy your food, but make sure you only eat when you're feeling hungry, and always stop when you're not feeling hungry anymore. I promise you – that's all you need to do.

Susan's tip:
I found my inner caveman

Hi, my name is Susan. I'm 22-years-old and I have lost 32lbs. I went from 164lbs to 132lbs. I did it by finding my inner caveman!

My story:

Yep, I was really put off by the name – why can't it be called Cave woman diet? I really don't want to look like a caveman, but I do like the idea of going back to nature and trying to eat as healthily as possible, but not if it involves a big beard, a hairy chest, and clubbing wild animals to death before I can eat.

My doctor mentioned the diet to me, and I shrugged and smiled in the surgery and said "yes, of course I'll try it", but obviously had no intention of doing anything of the sort. I needed to lose weight because my blood pressure was high (and my weight was too high ... and it had become increasingly clear that there was a link between the two highs!).

The doctor was talking about getting me onto pills to control my blood pressure. I said I didn't want to do this – I had a friend who'd taken blood pressure pills and ended up with terrible depression. I wanted to avoid that. So I knew I had to lose weight. He suggested the caveman diet, so I left the surgery, went home and researched it on the computer.

The thing that struck me about all the descriptions of the caveman diet was that it was a real common sense diet... a healthy approach to trying to lose weight. It seemed to have a very straight forward, logical backbone to it and easy rules to follow.

Nothing to do with calories or Pilates classes. You didn't have to sit there and wonder whether you could eat egg yolks on a Wednesday, protein on a Friday or drink alcohol after 11pm ...just eat as if you were a caveman!

For those of you who are wondering...this means eating natural, unprocessed foods – meat, fish, eggs, berries, nuts, veg – these are the foods that our body was designed to eat, and anything else we put inside ourselves makes us fat. At least that's the message I told myself to keep things simple. And it worked. I had a hellish first week, yearning for bread, cakes and pasta, but then that passed and I started to feel better about myself and much fuller than I had before.

Then, a really interesting thing happened; I had to go to a friend's wedding and I had a huge blow-out - I drank all day on an empty stomach, picking at high fat canapés, crisps and dips, and then having the biggest meal in the evening with tons of pudding and loads of cake, I drank way into the evening then we went for fish and chips on the way home. I felt like I was treating myself ... letting myself go from this diet I'd put myself on ... but, honestly, the next day I felt so bad it made me realise just how great I'd been feeling on the caveman diet.

It took me a couple of days before I felt myself again, and I haven't wanted to go out on a limb since. The weight has fallen off me. I feel happier, healthier, my senses are more alert ... I just feel brilliant. When I went back to the doctors, my blood pressure had dropped right down so I didn't need to take the blood pressure pills.

The thing that appealed to me about the diet was that it is not in the least complicated ... if you keep in your mind just to eat what a caveman would have eaten, that's all you have to do. So, you are in a restaurant and you are given the choice between fish and vegetables, and pasta carbonara ... you know which one the caveman would have been able to have - so have that (fish and vegetables!).

As well as being called the caveman diet, I've also seen this referred to as the clean diet. You are eating clean food (in other words -- foods that have not been processed or messed with). Cavemen wouldn't have been able to make coffee cake, donuts or Mississippi mud pie. But they would have been able to get hold of plenty of berries and nuts.

You might be reading this and thinking how dull this all sounds. I promise you it's far duller to be 30lbs overweight, and facing all the potential health hazard as well as high blood pressure. And it's easy - you have to just remember one thing - would a caveman have been able to eat this?

When cavemen ate it was to feed their bodies to keep themselves alive, and keep themselves as healthy as possible. That's not a bad premise for any diet.

Martin's tip:
Strict calorie control, but eating whatever I want

Hi, my name is Martin. I'm 30-years-old and I have lost 42lbs. I went from 246lbs to 204lbs. I did it by counting calories. It doesn't sound like much of a tip, but I think it's the easiest way to do it. Just be strict with yourself – give yourself a calorie target every day, and take it one day at a time. Don't worry about the long haul or what about Christmas, what about the summer holidays – just focus on the here and now, and making sure that every day you don't go over your calorie ceiling. If you do that, you will lose weight.

My story:

I know people say that calories aren't equal – there are good calories and bad calories – you are supposed to avoid calories with fat and sugar in, and eat calories with vitamins and protein. I know that, I really do, but it's very complicated trying to work out what you can and can't eat, and worrying what to order in a restaurant and turning into a madly fussy eater who only eats spinach. I found it much easier to set myself a daily calorie limit and stick to it.

I allowed myself 1500 calories a day, and that was it. I had 300 calories for breakfast (scrambled egg on toast, usually), 500 for lunch and 500 for dinner, and 200 for a drink or a snack. I just did that every day and I lost weight.

My gut feeling is that people complicate it too much. It all gets horribly difficult when you're told that avocados are fattening…but they're good for you. Nuts are full of goodness, but fattening. It's hellish to work out what you can and can't eat. I found it easier and straight forward to play the numbers game.

Let's face it, you can get fat from eating healthy food too. Count the calories – just do it, stick to it and the weight goes – problem solved.

READERS RESPONSES

Mandy B:
   Love your kitchen

Hi, my name is Mandy. I'm 60-years-old and I have lost 40lbs. I went from 190lbs to 150lbs. I did it by revisiting my whole approach to food, and cooking much more at home, so I knew exactly what was going into it, and by enjoying new flavours. So, basically, my tip is – learn to love your kitchen!

My story:

I lost weight properly when I fell in love with cooking, and being in my kitchen. It was only when I really started to get to grips with cooking for myself, and making tasty food that was low in fat and low calorie, that I managed to shift the weight.
   I think there were two psychological bonuses to preparing things for myself ... first of all, putting effort into cooking things properly for myself made me feel special when I was eating, and not as if I was denying myself tasty foods constantly. The second bonus came because I just became more aware, generally, of food and tastes. I

found that my taste in food changed and I wanted to eat healthier foods, foods that were better for me.

These were the key things I did –

1. I grew a herb garden. I know that sounds a bit dull, but if I was only eating salads, it was nice to have them with tons of coriander on them or home-grown mint and parsley. The mint was lovely for fresh mint tea. I grew chillies that were great for spicing up vegetable stew or rubbing onto chicken before grilling it to give it a bit of a tang.

2. I bought lemon and lime. I cut right down on the fruit I was eating because I was eating tons of it, and obviously it's full of sugar. I know it's good for you, but I was eating way too much. Lemons and limes had all the goodness without the sugar. I'd squeeze lemon into hot water to drink in the morning and use lemons and limes to flavour foods ... either by squeezing them, or grating the zest into dishes. I promise you it makes a real difference when you start cooking nice food for yourself, instead of buying diet versions of normal food. It's hard to feel looked after and cherished when you're buying frozen diet food. If you're chopping coriander, rubbing chilli on to chickens and squeezing lemons and limes into food it makes it all much more exciting and palatable.

3. I bought mustard and horseradish and, like I said earlier, grew my own chillies. The reason for these spicy foods is that they help any food that might otherwise be bland. When I grilled a whole load of vegetables, I would put a half teaspoon of horseradish into a cup with a few dessert spoons of boiling water mix it all up and pour it over the vegetables while they were grilling then I'd serve them on a bed of coriander and mint with a squeeze of lemon and it tasted absolutely gorgeous… full of taste (which I think also helps you feel full up which is why I would avoid all dull diet foods if I were you!!!)

4. I controlled the portions I was having. If I was eating things that may lead to me putting on weight, like pasta or potatoes, I was able to weigh them out or measure them out. The key to getting the right portion, is to have a portion the size of your fist, no bigger. When you go out to eat they will give you way too much food and it's

very hard not to eat it. Also, once you learn the whole concept of portion control no food is really off limits.

5. If you have a chicken breast, but don't want to eat all of it, slice it long ways rather than in half. I know this sounds daft - you are getting the same amount of food, but if you cut a chicken breast in half it looks like half. If you slice it down the middle it doesn't look as if you are cheating yourself out of half a breast of chicken. The same goes for a baguette... instead of having a short stumpy piece of bread have a longer piece but only half of it, then you feel as if you've had a proper meal.

6. I tried to buy vegetables that I have never tried before ... and seek out the freshest food around. I now go to a market on Saturday afternoons to buy loads of lovely fresh vegetables, in season, that hasn't been flown halfway around the world. I bought a coconut last night and had a go at cooking chicken and Coconut milk with chilli. By the time I added garlic, onion, broccoli and spinach, I had a huge bowl of comfort food that was really delicious with coriander sprinkled on the top. Honestly -- I promise you -- it's the way forward if you want to lose weight.

7. I bought spicy pepper blends which I sprinkled onto popcorn and other low calorie treats. The taste is there without the calories. It worked for me!

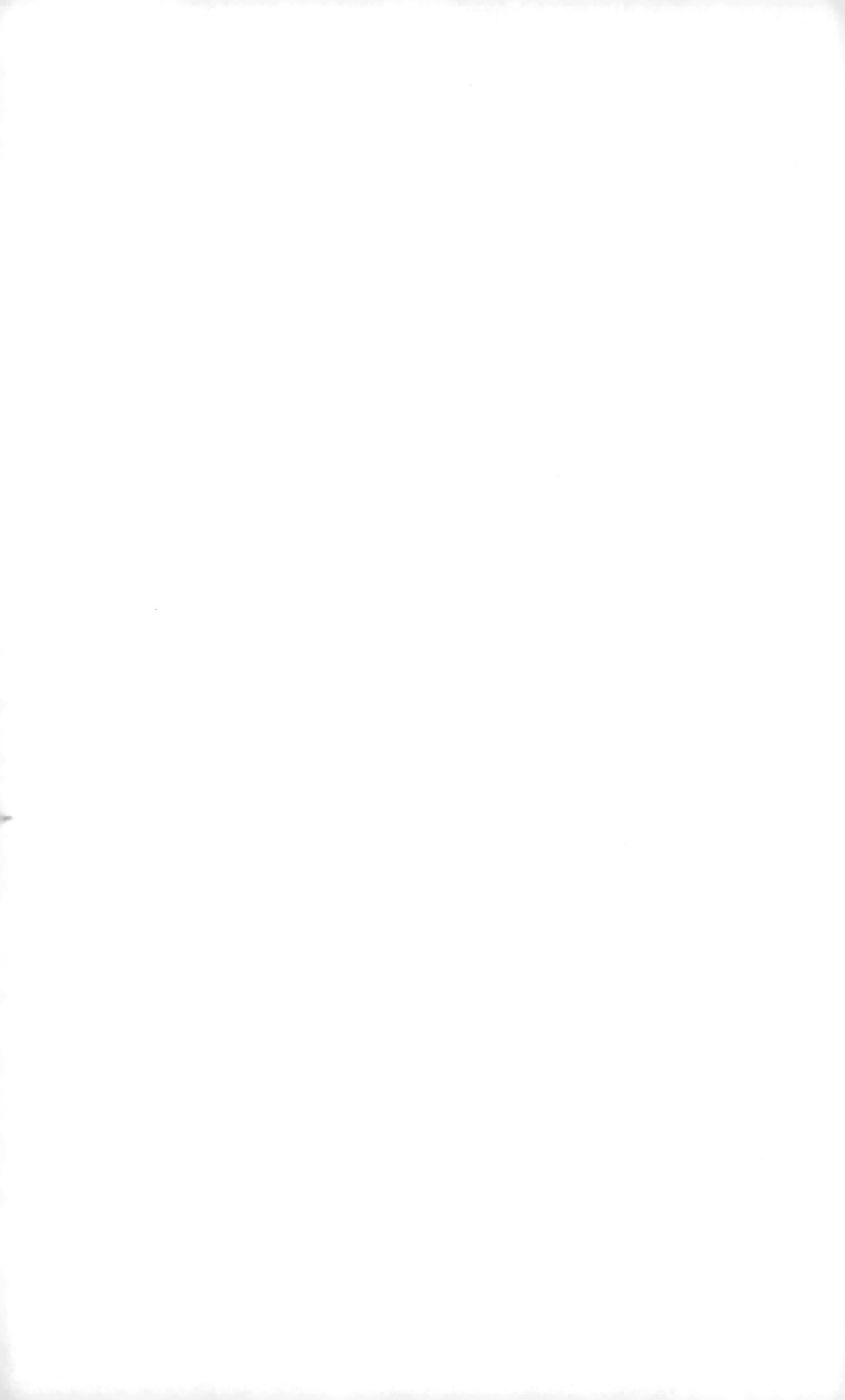

SECTION TWO

Psych yourself in instead of
psyching yourself out

PSYCHOLOGICAL ISSUES

This second section looks at the psychological issues involved in weight loss...how do you convince yourself not to eat when you really want to? How do you stop yourself from reaching for the crisps, cake, takeaways and break basket, when every fibre of your being urges you to do so?

For me, the way I coped, and broke the link between emotional well-being and eating was by repeating phrases to myself, like 'I only eat when I'm hungry', 'food is just to stop hunger' over and over and over until my emotions caught up with my voice. It will happen, and it will lead you to questioning what you're doing. If you bite into a big cream cake when you're not remotely hungry, while chanting 'I only eat when I'm hungry', a part of you will start to feel uncomfortable. You'll find yourself questioning what you're doing, and once you start questioning, the logical side of you will take over from the emotional side, and you'll find it easier to talk yourself out of eating all the time.

Certainly that was my experience. It was the experience of these people, too:

Claire's story: I did a psychological make-over

Hi, my name is Claire. I'm 42-years-old and I have lost 38bs. I went from 178lbs to 140lbs and I did it by sorting my head out! In short, I gave myself a psychological make-over. My tip to you is to do the same – you need to sort your head out if you're to have any chance of getting rid of that tummy!

My story:

My tip to you is to think very carefully about why it is that you have got fat. I know that sounds like a silly question - it might well be because you've eaten too much! But considering all the dangers of being overweight, why have you allowed this to happen? You might be shrugging at this point and thinking you'll skip over this section but please don't. Because I found that once I'd worked out what psychological problems I had that were leading me to eat too much, I was in a much better shape to sort out issues surrounding the amount I ate and drank.

I hope that doesn't sound too heavy, but I also used to be hopeless with money, socialise too much, and eat and drink way too much. When I stopped and did what I call a "psychological makeover" (PMO) I found myself much more in control ... not just with money and going out socialising all the time, but also with eating and drinking. I'd just lost control of my life, in so many ways, and desperately needed to get it back.

My psychological makeover came from spending time with a friend who had been an alcoholic, and had been in treatment, and knew what it took to get him off alcohol. He talked to me about the way in which his life was examined and analysed by those treating him, and the changes it led him to make. I took on board everything he told me about the course, and I worked out whether there were any lessons that I could learn from them. The answer was a very resounding – yes!

These are the things I did as part of my eight stage PMO:

dreams

mask
negativity
selfishness
stress
settling
waiting
laziness

Write them down, one below the other, with room to write alongside them, and jot notes about your own life as I explain. I promise this will help you.

Dreams - I wasn't being true to what my own dreams were. I'd always wanted to work in fashion, but I knew my parents would frown, so I had taken a job in a post office, then moved to a bank. I had a decent job, with a decent income, good work hours and friendly co-workers, but I wasn't living the dream I'd always had for myself. I knew I had to change this and live my life for me.

Mask - this ties into the first point really, but I discovered that I was showing the world what I thought they wanted to see - a professional, sensible, sophisticated woman with a good job in the bank. That wasn't me. I was effectively wearing a mask and being what I thought people wanted me to be rather than who I was.

Negativity - there's no doubt that there were a lot of negative people in my life, people who made me feel worse about myself when I spent time with them. I knew I had to cut them out.

Selfishness - I was living a selfish life, a life just for me. I changed things, and weaved in some charity work that made me feel much better about myself. Feeling more positive about myself, and confident in myself, was a key to making me want to treat myself better, and eat more healthily.

Stress - there's no doubt that I was really sweating the small stuff. Worrying about whether I'd put the bins out in the right place, had I told the milkman I wanted skimmed milk, did I remember to do things on time… stressing things that really didn't need to be stressed about. I knew I needed to relax, take a deep breath and learn to let go of things which really didn't matter that much.

Settling - is there anyone who hasn't done this one? I knew I was settling for a job I didn't like, in a relationship that had nothing to inspire me, and a life that didn't really fulfil me. I decided to try not to settle … even if it meant being on my own, that was better than settling for someone who I wasn't madly in love with.

Waiting -- I was very good at this! I kept saying I'd go onto a fashion design course, or start making my own clothes, or save up for a sewing machine, or go to the gym … tomorrow. I spent a lot of time waiting for tomorrow that never came. I've learnt that if something is worth doing is worth doing now. Just start, don't spend your life forever waiting.

Laziness - I realised that instead of feeling sorry for myself for being in a job I wasn't wildly keen on, I needed to get out there and change things. Things weren't going to change by themselves … whether that be my weight, my job, my life or my prospects. Don't be wishy-washy, vague and lazy. If you want it: go out and get it. If you change your life for the better, you'll find that everything will fall into place, and the need to eat will disappear and your motivation to get slim and healthy will appear.

Mike's tip: The three week watershed

Hi, my name is Michael. I'm 38-years-old and I have lost 50lbs. I went from 252lbs to 202lbs. I did it by eating smaller meals. I'd tried to lose weight loads of times before, and this time I was successful because I gave myself three weeks to get started. My tip is – if you can get yourself across the three week barrier, you can do it. Bear than in mind when you're on a diet, fed up and wanting to stop…keep going for three weeks!

My story:

I tried to lose weight … cutting out the pints of beer, the takeaways and the fried breakfasts, thinking about everything I ate, and trying to cut down to smaller, healthier meals. I was doing well for a week, then weighed myself and discovered I'd lost one pound. One pound!

It felt like a kick in the teeth. I'd dramatically altered the way I eat and all that happened was that I lost one pound. If things kept going on like this I wouldn't lose the weight I wanted to lose until I was about 120-years-old.

Needless to say, like 1 million people before me, I gave up, went back to the pub and back to my old ways. I enjoyed the takeaways and a few pints with my mates and decided I must be one of those people who just can't lose weight.

The way I broke the cycle of dieting for a short period of time, getting fed up, stopping, then doing the whole thing again, was when someone said to me that you have to give yourself time to get started. You have to do whatever you're going to do to lose weight for three weeks minimum before you come to a judgement on how it's going. Whatever you decide to do … whether it's Weight Watchers, the Cambridge diet, healthy eating, cutting back carbs, whatever it is - do it for three weeks before forming a view. You have to. The simple fact is - if you can't guarantee to do it for three weeks, you will not survive, because those first three weeks are crucial.

It takes a little while for the impact of what you are doing to register on the scales. It might register straightaway, like my one pound loss, or two pound loss, but that isn't enough incentive to keep going. I managed to crack it by not weighing myself for three weeks then when I got on the scales after three weeks I'd lost 7lbs. That was massively motivating, made me want to carry on, and reaffirmed that I was doing the right thing. The weight loss didn't carry on at that level, I had some good weeks and bad weeks, but I was able to endure it because I got those three weeks in at first so that my routine of weighing myself every Monday started with me already having lost seven pounds, so already feeling motivated.

I urge you to give yourself time. Don't do what I kept doing, and dieting for seven days expecting to see tremendous results, getting pissed off when there are no real changes, and falling back into old eating habits. It's taken quite a long time for you to put your weight on ... certainly with me it crept slowly over about three years - is it too much to expect that you give it three weeks of dieting to begin the process of getting rid of it?

So, just to repeat my psychological tip - decide what you're going to do – as I've said, I did it by cutting out all the things I knew were bad for me and having smaller meals - then give yourself three weeks before you judge it.

It's just three weeks ... you can do it.

Stick to it for three weeks then weigh yourself or measure yourself and come to a view. I think that 99% of people will have lost some weight after three weeks - enough weight for them to feel happy with the way the first three weeks have gone and inspire them to carry on.

The same theory applies when you're a few months into the diet, and you have a bad gym day, or a bad eating day, or you end up in the pub with your mates can't resist that fourth pint of beer... it took you years to put this weight on, one bad day isn't going to derail it. Shrug it off and get back on the bandwagon. No matter how badly you slip up, it doesn't matter, you've only lost control when you decide to lose control. You have it within you just shrug it off and carry on again.

Maria's story: I worked out the difference between emotional eating and eating for hunger.

Hi, my name is Maria. I'm 26-years-old and I have lost 34lbs. I went from 164lbs to 130lbs and I did it by realizing that I wasn't eating because I was hungry, but for emotional reasons. I identified when those times were, and I stopped doing it.

Note from Bernie: there were so many responses from people saying that the way they lost weight was to get control of their emotional eating that I have included two tips on coping with emotional eating. This is the first one ...

My story:

I was well aware that I was eating for emotional reasons, and not just because I was hungry. I was comfort eating. I'd reach out for food when things weren't right – when I was stressed, lonely or sad. The food made me feel immediately better, but, over the years, it had led to me putting on a lot of weight, which had the effect of making me feel more stressed, sadder and more lonely! I knew this in my head, but that didn't seem to make any difference to how I behaved...as soon as I was stressed, I ate. Worse than this, eating so much made me feel bad, so I'd eat more to overcome the bad feelings, and end up feeling even worse.

So, I was in the classic cycle of overeating. The trouble was that this was something I'd always done. I didn't think I'd ever be able to work out the difference between feeling hungry and wanting to eat, and feeling lonely, sad or fed up and wanting to eat. How would you ever know the difference? If there was food around, I wanted it. I knew that if my stomach rumbled I was hungry, but I wasn't aware of any other subtle signs about whether I was hungry or just eating for emotional reasons.

It was when I managed to distinguish between my emotional eating and my eating because I was hungry, that I made the breakthrough, and lost the weight. So my tip to any would-be dieters is: work out when you're eating for emotional reasons and when you are eating because you're hungry. Once you can do that, it's much easier to stop doing it.

So – how do you do it? This is what I did:

First of all, I wrote down everything I ate and how I was feeling when I ate. It started off simply - I had a bagel for breakfast, a cheese salad roll for lunch, then a packet of crisps Twix and more sandwiches at 4pm.

Why did I suddenly eat so much?

When I looked at what was happening, I realised that 4pm was the time that my husband phoned me and told me that he couldn't get back in time to pick our kids up from school. They have clubs til 5pm, so I would have to leave at 4:30pm to pick them up, meaning leaving work early. My instant response was to eat. Instead of saying to my husband "no, you promised you do it, you have to pick the children up," I rushed out and ate loads.

I was worried about letting my boss down by leaving early, worried about the kids, and annoyed at my husband. Without stopping to think, I filled the emotion and upset with food.

Most worryingly of all, as I kept the diary for a few weeks, I realised that eating was my primary emotional coping mechanism. If I became upset, lonely or bored, I'd eat. I'd eat when I felt stressed, carry on eating when I was full, and start eating whether I was hungry or not. Basically I was eating to feel better.

I felt hopelessly out of control around food, and once I started eating to fill emotional voids, I couldn't stop. I'd want to eat and eat and eat until I felt better. It was almost as if I was loading the food on top of the problems to stop them bothering me. I was creating a layer that separated me from the world. I loved the feeling that stuffing myself gave me, but I hated the feeling afterwards - the resentment, self-hatred, and anger at my lack of control. I had to learn to identify when I felt this emotional hunger, before I could begin to try not to eat.

It took quite a long time for me to work it all out, but these are the things I discovered along the way about the difference between emotional hunger and physical hunger.

§ First of all, physical hunger arrives gradually. You feel a little bit hungry, then a little bit more hungry until you are really quite peckish. Emotional hunger hits you like a thunderbolt; one minute you're fine, you get a negative phone call or have a negative thought and - boom - you've eaten three packets of chips before you can work out why you've done it.

§ When it comes to emotional hunger, you'll be driven to eat a certain type of food. I went carbohydrate crazy... not sweet things, but big jacket potatoes stuffed with loads of cheese and coleslaw, pizza, chips, takeaways ... if you are truly physically hungry, you are not anywhere near as particular about the sort of food you want - an apple, a piece of bread - they are all fine. Emotional hunger demands a particular sort of comfort food.

§ Emotional hunger is out of control ... you can't say to yourself that you'll have a couple of chips - the whole lot has gone. I found that I didn't even really enjoy the taste of the food, I hadn't really noticed I was eating it, I was just shoving it inside myself to make myself feel better.

§ The key thing that I've found with emotional hunger vs physical hunger was that emotional hunger was never satisfied ... I'd keep eating and eating and eating way beyond feeling comfortable and I'd want to keep eating as much as I could.

§ Emotional hunger isn't located in the stomach. Rather than a growling belly or a pang in your stomach, you feel your hunger as a craving you can't get out of your head.

§ Emotional hunger often leads to regret, guilt, or shame. When you eat to satisfy physical hunger, you're unlikely to feel guilty or ashamed because you're simply giving your body what it needs. If you feel guilty after you eat, it's likely because you know deep down that you're not eating for nutritional reasons.

So my tip is to identify all the times you eat for emotional reasons. Use a food diary, and think about all the points I've listed above. After that, you need to work out how to stop your emotional eating. I admit that I did it by joining the lighter life program - a very low calorie weight loss program which a lot of people don't agree with. I found it was useful for me to take all the food out of my diet so I wasn't around food, couldn't think about food, and dismissed it from my life. Simultaneously, the lighter life people talk to you about how to gain control around food. The whole thing really worked for me, and I feel much happier now, but when I look back at the craziness I used to have when I was around food it's almost like someone on drugs looking for their next fix - it meant everything to me to get the sort of food I wanted and to eat it quickly until I was so full I was almost sick. Obviously, if you feel like I did, you might want to see your GP or a psychiatrist to talk through the issues. But the first thing to do is just to be clear and honest with yourself about whether you are eating for emotional reasons rather than physical. Good luck.

(The second emotional eating story)

Patricia's story: I stopped my emotional eating

Hi, my name is Pat. I'm 46-years-old and I have lost 48lbs. I went from 208lbs to 160lbs and I did it by realizing that I wasn't eating because I was hungry, but for emotional reasons. The big thing I did which allowed me to lose weight, was to stop my emotional eating. Now, I know that doesn't sound like much of a tip ... of course we all know we could lose weight if we stopped our emotional eating, but what I did that I'd like to pass on to you as my number one tip, is that I identified exactly how, why, and when I fell into patterns of emotional eating. Once I'd done that, getting some sort of control over my food intake was quite straightforward. And after that, losing weight was much easier.

I suppose I knew I was an emotional eater because I was eating way too much, way beyond the point of satisfying hunger, stuffing myself with food for the sake of it. But I didn't realise that it was called "emotional hunger" and I just thought I was insanely greedy, and couldn't work out why. I'd be getting on with my life, then somehow I'd be overwhelmed by this need to eat, or a thought would enter my mind and that was it ... I couldn't relax until I'd eaten something, and not just something, loads and loads of food until I felt so completely full up I couldn't move - really fattening food - all the sorts of foods that anyone with a weight problem would work really hard to stay away from. I felt completely out of control around these foods, and compelled beyond all common sense to eat and eat and eat. I simply had to eat.

I didn't feel able to do anything about the fact that I ate until I could understand why I did it. I didn't know why this was happening. Like I say, I thought of myself as being greedy which just made me feel worse than ever. Then, I realised that what I was doing was emotional eating, and worked out a way to stop it.

My story:

I began by going to see my GP, because I went to join the gym and discovered by their measuring and weighing techniques that I was "morbidly obese". I was definitely obese, but didn't really think of myself as being really huge, and I think part of me always thought that I could do something about this if I really tried. Hence my attempts to join a gym. The people in the gym were lovely, but said they would feel much happier if I went to see my GP first, just to check that he was happy for me to start an exercise program. When I went to see my GP and started talking to him, he asked me what sort of food I ate in the day, and I replied, quite honestly, that in a normal day I might have fruit and cereal for breakfast, a sandwich or jacket potato for lunch, and then usually a salad or jacket potato in the evening. He looked at me above his half-moon glasses and raised his eyebrows.
"Can I be honest with you?" he asked me.
"Of course," I replied.
"You wouldn't be this size if you ate like that," he said.
That's when I explained to him that the food intake I had described was a normal day, but that there were lots and lots of very abnormal days when I went absolutely ballistic around food. He leaned over and touched my arm, and said "why do you think you eat like this?" that's when I burst into tears, and said I didn't know.
I have no idea why I burst into tears, and I was madly embarrassed at having done so, but looking back at that moment now, four years on, and having lost over 45lbs, it was the best moment of my life. He got me to explain to him how disciplined I could be with food, but then sometimes, for no reason at all, I'd go absolutely mad and need to eat gross amounts of fatty food. He said he thought this was emotional eating, and whilst it would be useful for me to start on a

diet and exercise program, I also needed to take a good look at the emotions that were causing me to eat. He recommended a psychologist.

I'm crying as I'm writing this, because the truth is that the psychologist he sent me to see changed my whole life. If you think you may have the same issues that I have, I'd recommend going to talk to your GP. He can put you in touch with a psychologist on the NHS... in the meantime, read on, and I'll tell you how it all worked for me.

I turned up at the psychologist's office feeling a bit of an idiot ... I didn't know what she was going to ask me, or what I was going to say. I didn't have any big worries or issues. My parents haven't split up, I haven't lost my job, I didn't have any real money worries. I was just this fat girl who couldn't stop eating.

She made it very clear that she thought there were underlying issues related to my need to eat in such large quantities. We talked about the whole thing, and in my instance she became very clear that it was my inability to have proper relationships with men that caused a great void in my life which I was filling with food. We did a lot of talking about past relationships, and things that had gone very wrong in them, and I continue to see her to talk about all these issues. But she was very keen to help me as quickly as possible with the overeating, so she helped me to try and work out what the triggers were for me to overeat.

She explained that most emotional eating is linked to unpleasant feelings, but it can also be through positive emotions. Some people eat too much when they're feeling very happy, because they feel relaxed and happy and want to continue the happiness, and reward themselves for the lovely feelings they have.

It soon became clear that this wasn't what I was doing. It was unpleasant feelings that made me eat too much. After much talking, thinking, and analysing, it became clear that I was feeling sadness, anxiety and loneliness, and that was what was forcing me to eat.

She said that I was numbing myself with food ... avoiding emotions I'd rather not feel. This might not be what you are doing ... other people eat when they are stressed. Apparently there is a biological reason for this – cortisol is the stress hormone released when you feel worried or under pressure, and this triggers cravings for foods which give you a burst of energy. If you feel like stress in your life is completely out of control, you may feel that the eating you do to compensate is equally out of control. I want to emphasise that I'm not a psychologist -- I'm just telling you my story about what I learnt when I tried to take control of my over-eating. The other thing that can cause emotional eating is boredom or feelings of emptiness ... filling a void in your life. It occupies you, and distracts you from any dissatisfaction you may be feeling.

There are other, bigger issues, of course. People can start overeating when a parent dies, or they go through a traumatic experience. In my view the only way you are going to work out what it is that forces you to overeat is to keep the most detailed emotional eating diary you possibly can or to talk to a psychologist. You need to try and work out what the patterns are behind your emotional eating. They might be really subtle.

One thing that provoked a turnaround in my understanding of my eating was when I had a complete binge after chatting to a friend on the phone, and she said she had to go. I felt immediate emptiness and loneliness (except that I didn't, of course, because I stuffed these emotions down by eating everything I could find in the fridge). It's not always big dramatic events that throw you off course, but little things, like when you're chatting to a friend, and she has to go. Her saying she was going seemed like a rejection and it triggered this descent into mad eating.

I kept details of how I felt, what I wanted to eat and what I actually ate.

I found I would stuff myself with food when I went to family functions, or when I was facing a big night out with more glamorous friends. On many occasions, I got off the train to go to a social function, headed straight into a kebab shop, bought myself tons of food, and then just got the train back home without going to the function. Why was I doing that? What was I scared of? It seemed to all come back to worrying about relationships with men.

It helped me enormously simply being able to identify these emotions. Then I had to try and kick the habit of going from that emotion to eating. I did that surprisingly simply. The psychologist said that a lot of people have a lot of problems breaking the link, but I found that by doing things like putting my feet flat on the floor and breathing deeply for a minute, or getting on the phone to another friend, helped enormously.

For me, the tip that led to my massive weight loss was finding out what it was that made me overeat. The rest seem to take care of itself. If you find yourself in the position I was in, or if any of this resonates with you, I wish you lots and lots of luck. You can make yourself feel much better, lose the weight, and start to have a happier life. Go down to your GPs and see whether anyone there can help you. Lots of luck and lots of love.

Charlie's story: Get a reality check

Hi, my name is Charlie. I'm 28-years-old and I have lost 56lbs. I went from 182lbs to 126lbs and I did it by grabbing my life by the horns and sorting myself out. Brutal, but effective!!

My story:

My tip for losing weight is quite brutal -- I know this will sound very hard and difficult, but it is: get a reality check. That's my tip to you – get a reality check.

I was very overweight (I'm only 4'10"), but kind of lying to myself about just how big I was. I avoided mirrors, kept away from people taking photographs, and never got on the scales. It allowed me to think that actually things weren't too bad, but the truth is that if you are avoiding looking in full-length mirrors, and diving out the way anytime anyone pulls a camera out, you might not be dealing with reality!

My reality check moment came at a wedding ... no place for escape. When I was told that I had been picked to be a bridesmaid, my first thought was "no no no no no" there's absolutely no way I can walk down the aisle in a dress with everyone looking at me. But then another part of me reassured me that I could easily lose weight in time for the wedding, and actually it might be quite a good thing to have a function that I really wanted to lose weight for ... it might give me the motivation I need to lose weight.

So, I accepted the kind invitation, and put off the first bridesmaid fitting thinking that if I could delay it a bit, I could lose weight. It didn't happen. So in the end I had to go along and have the bridesmaid dress fitting. I shut my eyes and put my hand over my ears as they did the measuring, and refused to look directly into the mirror. This continued throughout the process of preparing for the wedding, but on the wedding day I put my bridesmaid dress on, not having lost any weight at all, and walked down the aisle after my friend – a little ball waddling along behind her.

That was all fine ... no mirrors in church, no need for me to face how big I had got. But then came the real horror, and the moment when I got the biggest reality check of all - the photos came back from the wedding. I was huge. I mean it. I was literally twice the width of one of the other bridesmaids. I really was enormous. It was the reality check I needed, because even though I'd been aware that I was overweight, I hadn't taken it really seriously. As I looked at myself I realised that this wasn't just about losing a couple of pounds to fit into a smaller bridesmaid's dress, I had a real problem. I had to get myself back into shape because the size I was in those pictures was very unhealthy.

That shocking moment forced me to take weight loss much more seriously than I had done ever before. I weighed myself and discovered that I was 182lbs (I was convinced that I was around 150lbs), then I took a good look at myself in the mirror, and looked at the clothes I was wearing - all of them baggy, designed not for their beauty or flattering nature, but to cover me up. How had I let this happen?

The truth is that I had let this happen by ignoring the facts. I wasn't dealing with reality. My tip to you is to look in the mirror and get on the scales, get yourself a measured, and deal with the truth of the size that you are. Don't lie to yourself. It's much harder to commit yourself to lose weight and to do all you can to get fit and healthy, if you're refusing to acknowledge how overweight you are in the first place. I'm sorry if this all sounds brutal, but I do think a lot of us choose to ignore the signs, and make life doubly hard for ourselves by avoiding reality.

In the end, after my shock reality check, I managed to lose the weight by making small changes. I cut out sugar to start with.... I let myself eat what I wanted, but only things without sugar. The next thing I did was cut out white foods -- particularly pasta, bread, biscuits and potatoes. By this time I was starting to lose weight, so felt motivated to stick to it. Then someone mentioned to me that alcohol has a lot of sugar in it, so I decided to try and cut right down on that. Instead of having wine, I had vodka and tonic, first of all because wine comes in a bottle, and once I've got it open I can't stop, and also because vodka and tonic has less sugar in it.

I kept doing that – cutting back on the bad things gradually, until I was eating a really healthy diet, then I introduced exercise, and the weight just drifted away. I had a few plateaus, of course, and I managed to fight through those, and I had a lot of moments where I almost slipped, and moments when I actually slipped - having fish and chips and half a bottle of wine, but I managed to get back onto the diet again the next day. I never kidded myself that I was only losing a couple of pounds - I knew I had a lot of weight to lose, and I knew it was important that I lost it. It was this honesty with myself and facing up to the reality that enabled me to finally lose the weight for good.

SECTION THREE:

Be nice to yourself; treat yourself with respect

BE NICE TO YOURSELF

I think this is a much misunderstood area of weight loss. People who are overweight beat themselves up every day, they feel bad about themselves and wish they didn't look the way they do. Overeating and lack of control around food are desperately difficult to deal with because food is available around us all the time...we can't get away from it. I don't wish the belittle those who have drug or alcohol problems, but dealing with those issues means abstaining from them...food is very different. You have to eat; there is no choice. That means that you have to operate around food all the time, deciding what to eat. If you make bad decisions, you beat yourself up, but unlike an alcoholic who might sall off the wagon every few months, you have the propensity to fall off it every five minutes because food is in and around us all the time. It means you're beating yourself up and feeling awful all the time.

There's also the fact that overeating shows itself so clearly. You look fat and feel uncomfortable so you feel furious with yourself. Your way to cope with feeling furious has been to eat, so you then want to eat which makes you feel worse and more and more fed up.

Well - don't worry. Relax. The world hasn't ended. If you're jeans are tight it's not the end of the world. Just stop, breath and don't call yourself horrible names.

You've got this. Here are some techniques for feeling better when the world around you feels pretty horrible.

Sonia's tip: Meditation

Hi, my name is Sonia. I'm 39-years-old and I have lost 32lbs. I went from 170lbs to 138lbs. I did it by going to Weight Watchers. I found it quite stressful keeping an eye on everything I was eating and counting up the points, and kept getting fed up, stressed out and giving up. Then, I'd find some motivation from somewhere and start again, but the same thing would happen – I'd get fed up with it, miss a few weeks, and stop. In the end I managed to stick to it for one reason, and I'll share that with you now. I've lost most of the weight (I've got around 7lbs to go). And the thing I did? I started meditating.

My story:

I was about 40lbs overweight and fed up with life. I couldn't think of a way of losing weight, because every time I tried, I gave up. Nothing seemed to motivate me. I found I'd had the best luck with Weight Watchers, so I decided to try that again. I began well, as I always do, but then started to get fed up, stopped doing it for a few days, and never got back on it. I just didn't feel I had control over my food intake…eventually the food would win!

I'd be great for a couple of weeks then would wreck all my days of good dieting by suddenly eating a load of food, or drinking a load of alcohol, even if I wasn't hungry, and that was it – diet over, all ruined.

I remember one time when I'd been really good for couple of weeks, eating healthily, and going for regular walks, and cutting out the pub visits, then I had a really tough day at work, ran to catch the train home and just missed it. The next one wasn't for 40 minutes, and before I'd thought it through, I was in the fish and chip shop eating a huge bag of chips and curry sauce while I was waiting. Once I was three quarters of the way through it, I decided I wanted more, so went to the newsagents and bought a chocolate bar, then went to the pub and had two large glasses of wine. I then got on the train, feeling really sick, and just desperately confused about what it was made me do that. I wasn't hungry. I wasn't planning to eat, but it was as if one little knock-back had ruined everything. If the train had come into the platform, I'd have just got on it, but the disappointment and annoyance of missing the train just made me lash out and reach for food and drink.

And it wasn't as if I could stop myself – it was almost as if I had the food and had eaten it before I realised what I was doing. I seemed to be suddenly in the fish and chip shop and then halfway through a large packet of chips before I had even thought about whether I was hungry. The more I thought about it, I realised that incidents like this were quite common – I was out of control.

Realising this came at the same time as I saw a leaflet about mindfulness and meditation, and it had the simple message "get control of your life again". It struck me that that was exactly what I needed to do ... so I went along and learned to meditate.

Anyone who's not tried it, I would strongly advise it ... either download a YouTube video, get a book, or if you see classes on, go along and try it out.

It's not weird and wacky men in orange suits wailing and chanting – it's just a bunch of stressed out people who feel their lives are running away from them and want to get control.

The main thing that meditating did for me was to teach me to stop and think before doing things. It's given me the ability to pause for just a second, which makes all the difference. I can close my eyes and clear my mind of all the mad thoughts, breathe, and be more logical, less emotional.

I'm more relaxed and happier. I feel more in control and I've stopped using food as an emotional crutch. It takes a bit of practice, but I started by doing it in bed for five minutes at nights, and in the morning for five minutes before I get up. It helps me to clear my mind.

I seem to have more clarity and an emotional balance which, certainly for me, has helped me to be much more sensible about healthy food choices, and has led to me losing all the weight I wanted to.

Anyway – that's my tip. And my big, big message to you is to give it a go. We all know that answer to weight loss is in the mind, so why not just spend 10 minutes a day de-cluttering the mind and helping yourself enormously to live a healthy, happy life. Good luck!

Anna's tip: Get positive

Hi, my name is Anna. I'm 48-years-old and I have lost 50lbs. I went from 225lbs to 175lbs. I did it by getting positive and starting to like myself. Sounds a bit wishy-washy but I worked out that I was over-eating to make myself a happy person. I made the conscious decision to be a happy person, and losing weight was easier. Sounds odd? Read on...it's free and it worked for me!

My story:

One of the things that I found really hard about losing weight, was that everything was negative ... you couldn't eat this, you couldn't eat that...that was banned, this was banned. No alcohol, no biscuits with tea...ahhhh...it was all just so incredibly negative.

I had so much weight to lose, but it just felt like a horrible endless negative road stretching out ahead of me. So I gave up. I couldn't face the months, years of denying myself.

I think a lot of people give up because of this reason - you just get fed up with punishing yourself constantly with no obvious results or benefits from it. When you've got 50lbs to lose, shifting two or three a week doesn't feel like you're making much of a dent in the problem.

The way things changed for me was when I suddenly started to decide to be really positive about it all. I know this sounds a bit naff, and new age, but let me explain it like this...

I've always been really bad with money, hopeless at saving (very good at spending), and would never have a very good grip on my finances. I was mortgaged up to my eyeballs, and resented paying it every month for a small house in a very average area. Then one day I went on to Zoopla - the website that tells you how much your house is worth, and I discovered that my house had gone up in value by 12% since I bought it. In that instant I suddenly saw my whole mortgage payments in a much more positive light ... my house was actually worth a decent amount of money ... things weren't that bad. I suddenly became more interested in paying as much of the mortgage off as possible, and became good at saving money rather than spending it, because I wanted to get that mortgage paid off because I suddenly felt more positive and excited about my financial situation.

Exactly the same thing happened with weight loss -- I resented going to the gym, I resented the fact that I wasn't losing much weight, I resented having to cut back foods that I enjoyed ... I just resented everything. Then I went to the gym one time and the woman on reception said "blimey you look great -- you look like you've lost a lot of weight." I'd only lost about seven pounds, but I can't tell you what difference that comment made to me in that moment.

Suddenly I saw the whole thing in a much more positive light. At the gym that day I was determined to run further and exercise harder than I ever have before, and I came home and didn't fancy eating anything unhealthy I wanted to eat things were good for me because I'd enjoyed that moment of positivity. It was exactly the same feeling that I'd had with my house, when I discovered it was worth more than I expected. Positivity is an amazing thing!

Weight-wise, that comment changed everything for me ... suddenly losing weight had gone from a negative to a positive thing. From then on I arrived at the gym feeling good because someone had noticed that I looked better, this meant me wanting to go to the gym more often which led to me losing more weight and toning up further and more good comments, and it all spiralled in a very positive way and allowed me to lose a lot of weight. I've lost 50lbs and I've never felt better.

If I were to give people one reason why I managed to lose the weight it's because I got myself into a positive frame of mind about weight loss ... I started to look at healthy food as being good, and was excited at the fact that I got through a day without eating any rubbish, because it would make me look good in the end, and make me healthier. There is no doubt, for me, that the random comment by a woman whose name I still don't know, made a massive difference, because she hit me with something positive when I felt that everything was very negative. So my advice to you would be to try your hardest to look at your weight loss in a really positive way ... think of all the good things that will come out of it, don't think about the pain of exercising, think about how fabulous you going to look.

Look at the tuna salad you are about to eat, and instead of thinking -- I wish I had a Chinese takeaway -- just think about how much good it is doing you, how much better you are going to feel in the long run, and how amazing you are to be doing this for yourself. Surround yourself with positive people, and read positive things. Watch positive, uplifting videos on You Tube, and the great sports quotes which offer motivational tips. Just read them, read them again and don't allow any negativity to creep in. Keep that positivity up and when you start to lose the weight and start to feel better, you'll end up on the same cycle - feeling positive about weight loss and managing, finally, to shed the unwanted pounds properly and get yourself to a much healthier weight.

Kate's tip: Be nice to yourself

Hi, my name is Kate. I'm 67-years-old and I have lost 30lbs. I went from 170lbs to 140lbs. I did it by strict calorie counting. It wasn't easy, but I found it got much easier when I started being nice to myself.

My story:

I'm sure this must look like an odd tip to give you, but by being nice to yourself I mean respect yourself as much as anything. If you are eating too much and have put on weight, you may have given yourself the wrong impression that you're doing this because you're treating yourself to nice food, takeaways and dinner out. The way I lost weight is by learning that I wasn't treating myself nicely by filling myself with food. This was not a nice way to treat myself - it was cruel, heartbreaking and led to me being disappointed, sad and lonely. When I was feeling fat and horrid I didn't want go out and see my friends, I felt ashamed and sad. Is there anyone on earth who would describe putting yourself in this position as being nice to yourself?

No.

It's horrible.

Listen to me – I'm telling you – filling yourself with food is not 'being nice to yourself'. It's not. If you're doing that, you need to stop. Don't beat yourself up, don't have horrible voices in your head telling you how awful you are that you need to eat to feel better. Just stop doing it. Think of it as being nice to yourself, because that's what it is.

My tip is to think about the things you can do today that will make the 'you' of tomorrow much happier. Maybe it's walking a mile a day, maybe it's cutting out sugar, fat, going to Weight Watchers, whatever you want to do to lose the weight – own it, and smile at it. The mind-set I adopted was that this was for me… I wasn't punishing myself, I was looking after myself.

I lost weight through calorie counting, and by going to Zumba classes at the gym. I joined a diet group, and when I first started going, I hated the lady who ran it, who would preach at me and all the others there and tell us what we could and couldn't eat. Then I hated the Zumba teacher who shouted at us to jump higher skip higher, put more effort into it.

But then I had a mind-set change and I realised that all these people wanted me to be a happier person. They weren't doing it to upset me, or cause me grief. It was only my own head doing that.

So I decided to be nice to myself and to believe everyone else was being nice to me…and it worked. Feeling better and happier genuinely worked.

When I went to Zumba and they told me to work harder, I convinced myself it was because they wanted me to be the best possible version of myself. And when the diet group leader went on and on about vegetable soup I stopped thinking "shut up, leave me alone" and I started thinking - she's giving me this advice because she really cares and knows it really works.

I started realising that the people who were giving me weight watching advice were trying to treat me properly, and the voices in my head telling me to have another cake, and not worry about it, and to dismiss these experts, were not treating me properly. The voices had to change, not my efforts to lose weight.

Obviously, it would have been much easier to stop going to diet club and stop going to Zumba and sit at home eating cakes, but once I'd made that mental transition, that it was important for me to be nice to myself and that being nice to myself involved doing things that were good for my health, the motivation grew and grew and the weight started to fall off.

There were hiccups along the way, of course – an unexpected meal out with friends when I ate too much and drank too much, but I didn't beat myself up - every time my diet and exercise plan went wrong, I just resumed the diet the next day. Don't be afraid of failure, don't beat yourself up when you fail, smile and remember that the most important thing is to treat yourself properly.

Paul:
I got my self-esteem back.

Hi, my name is Paul. I'm 62-years-old and I have lost 78bs. I went from 248lbs to 170lbs and I did it by getting my self-esteem sorted.

There is no doubt that there is a link between how you feel about yourself and how you treat yourself. If you feel confident, happy and outgoing, then you eat foods that make you feel confident, happy and outgoing. Similarly, if you're feeling low and depressed and fed up, you reach for foods that will exacerbate that feeling. If you're in the cycle of feeling rubbish and eating rubbish, you've got to do something to get out of it. You've got to try and eat better and exercise more to make yourself feel better to get yourself into the positive cycle. As we all know (or why would you bought this book?) that's much easier said than done. You have probably tried dieting, as I had, tried exercising, as I had, and couldn't get out of the negative cycle. So, you could try doing what I did - I turned the cycle on its head, and decided to start treating myself better in the hope that that would make me eat better. It worked!

Remember just how much our emotional state impacts upon our physical state. Even the word disease comes from dis-ease... feeling dis at ease with ourselves. Emotional state is really important to your physical state, and that can depend on the environment you are in, the people you're socialising with, the stress you're under, how happy you are, how secure you are and how fulfilled you feel. I felt as if my self-esteem was really low, so I set about doing these six things, and challenging myself in these six areas, which put me in a better frame of mind to focus on getting myself superslim and superfit. And it worked – big time! I've lost over 75lbs.

So, these are the questions I asked myself:

Do I have a low self-esteem?

The easiest way to work this out is to describe yourself in a couple of sentences to an imaginary person in front of you. Do this now before reading any further on. OK. Done that? Then write down the adjectives you used when you described yourself.

This is a sentence that I used: "I'm a fat middle-aged man who is balding, lazy, gets lonely, but is quite nice to his friends."

I didn't realise how low my self-esteem was before I did this test, but experts think that the first words you use to describe yourself are very telling in terms of how you feel about yourself. I know this sounds a bit naff and hippyish, but I made myself look into the mirror every morning and say positive things about myself, reversing the sentences I had used to describe myself.

Horrible head chat

The second thing I made myself do was to talk about myself nicely. You know we all do that thing where we make a simple mistake and in our heads we say "you absolute idiot, what the hell are you doing, can't you do anything right?" Well, I fought very hard to stop it. As soon as I heard myself criticizing myself or putting myself down, I'd tell myself off. Indeed I wrote SHHC on my hand to remind myself to stop the horrible head chat. You can feel it coming on and you can stop it if you try. It doesn't happen at first, but if you keep trying you will stop it and you will feel a whole lot happier and nicer once it goes away.

Accept yourself

You are what you are, and you cannot change how you are in this instant. All you can do is make little changes to improve yourself for the future. But right now there is nothing you can do besides accept who you. In particular, try to accept the vulnerable or not-so-pretty parts of yourself; everyone has these; for example, it is not bad to be anxious or sad sometimes. If you hate walking into a crowded room, don't beat yourself up. Work on conquering the problems, but never think they make you bad or somehow less than other people.

Accept your bad bits as well is your good bits

No one is all good. Don't believe that for a minute. We are all made up of 1 million different bits and pieces - some of the bits are good and some other bits are bad. If you let yourself be defined by the bad bits you'll feel horrible. Think of all the good things you do... the friendships you have, the kindness you show your pets, the way in which you have managed to plant a lovely garden, keep the house clean and tidy. There are lots and lots of good things. We are more than a sum of the bad things, so focus on the good stuff too.

Don't just take criticism

I don't think you should ignore criticism, in fact you should be able to take criticism, but you should always exercise your own judgement when someone criticizes you. Separate criticism out into criticism that is valid, not valid, semi-valid and irrelevant. Make sure you just respond to the valid criticism only, and don't sink into a packet of chips if people criticise you unfairly – tell them.

Treat yourself as if you matter

How on earth are you supposed to eat properly, exercise properly and look after yourself if deep down within your psychology you think you're worthless? Make sure you encourage yourself to do the things you want to do, and give yourself time to be happy and nurtured. It's not your job to run-around making sure everyone else is happy all the time. You matter too!! Whether it's shovelling leftovers into your mouth, rushing around to make sure you're never late for anyone, or dashing to get everything ready for everyone else leaving you only half ready ... whatever it is (mothers be particularly aware - your kids are important but you matter too!!!!), look after yourself. I mean that. You've probably been over-eating for a reason. Take it from me - as someone who went through this and came out the other side - you are worth more than left-overs, second place and scraps!!!! No one in the world is more important than you. You are precious. Look after yourself.

Smile, count your blessings & don't worry.

Being overweight is tough…it affects every part of your life, but worrying about it isn't going to help. In fact, worrying about it is going to make everything much harder for you. Stress can paralyse you and thwart all your chances of losing weight.

So – smile, think of three wonderful things in your life, then go for a 10 minute walk.

That's all. You can easily build-up…just do one small thing to get started

Take it slowly, enjoy life, and SMILE.

SECTION FOUR

WAW! Water and walking

WALKING AND WATER

This section is simple, straightforward but vital. There are two things that I really want you to do when you're on your diet campaign - the first is to walk as much as you possibly can, the second is to drink as much water as possible. I'm not saying that you can never have wine and you have to walk everywhere. I'm saying just do as much of it as you possibly can. Try to have a small bottle or glass of water on your desk all the time, and try to make yourself get up and walk around...even for 10 minutes. If you can walk to work instead of driving - great - but even if it's just a walk around the office or to the end of the garden. Do as much as you possibly can.

Water is vital to fill you up and make you feel satisfied, and walking will make you feel better, healthier and as if you are looking after yourself. I promise you: if you do these two things, you WILL feel better and look better.

Water

Some of the readers who have contacted me have spoken about how important water was when they started listening to their bodies and only eating when they were hungry. Often they found they were thirsty rather than hungry. It also filled them up after exercising so they didn't feel the need to eat. A lot of the exercisers spoke about the difficulty of exercising and then being starving afterwards and wanting to eat, thus undoing some of the good work of the exercise. Drinking lots of water helped a great deal with this.

Some of the people I spoke to talked about feeling more alert when they had drunk water, and not getting headaches that they had been getting. Their energy levels lifted and their skin improved. Having improved skin might not necessarily lead directly to weight loss, but as you read through the tips in this book, you'll realise that many successful weight losers state "feeling good" as an important part of what enabled them to shift the weight.

It's important to remember that water makes up almost 70% of our bodies, with some of our internal organs containing even more (the liver is almost all water – some 95%, and remember the liver is responsible for breaking down fatty acids and transporting them to the blood so looking after the liver is important in weight loss. If you don't drink enough water, your liver cannot function properly to metabolise fat and remove toxins from the system).

So from a health perspective it is very important to take a lot of water in. Water also has the job of taking nutrients around the body. If you're cutting back on the food you're eating, you really want the nutrients you take in to be used properly by your body. Water does this, as well as acting as a catalyst for water soluble vitamins.

There is also the odd fact that drinking water helps get rid of water retention. The body retains water when it doesn't get enough of it, so as you start drinking more water your body will let go of the water it has been storing. You notice this in puffy faces and ankles.

The amount of water you should consume every day does vary depending on your height weight and fat loss goals, but as a ballpark figure you should be aiming for a gallon of water a day (so – around eight pints – which sounds a lot, but give it a go and see how many you can manage – any increase is good, and will help). That means a couple of glasses in the morning, a glass before each meal, and a few other glasses scattered through the day.

The other thing about drinking water, is that it stops you from having drinks that are no good for you: fizzy drinks, milky drinks and alcoholic drinks have a lot of sugar and/or fat in them that you can eliminate if you opt for water instead.

This isn't a secret tip or anything, but I pass it on to you because it's a fact that every single person I spoke to who had lost a lot of weight, said they had upped their intake of water considerably.

Walking

Walking is a great way to get light exercise and fresh air. Walking helps you to relax and calm down. Walking is good for your sanity. Go walking – do yourself a favour. Everyone who lost the weight spoke about the value of walking a lot.

This is what some of my readers thought:

Jane.
Re-think exercise

I'm 25-years-old and I have lost 30lbs. I went from 160lbs to 130lbs. I did it by cutting out unhealthy carbs. Like everyone else in the whole wide world, I found it hard to do, and I failed many times before I succeeded. The difference between the failures and the successful weight loss was one thing – exercise.

My story:

Like lots of women, I never liked exercise. I always thought of it as such a pain – not just the running around bit, but the getting changed in a crowded changing room, then the showering, drying hair, getting changed afterwards.

When I put on weight after my baby was born, I couldn't think of anything worse than taking my huge, fat body into the gym! I was 21, massively overweight, and with a baby to look after. Weight loss was a distant dream.

So, I cut back on unhealthy foods, and some weight started to come off, but I wasn't really committed to it...I'd have some good days, some bad days.

A friend said that by exercising I'd speed up the weight loss, and I'd look better because I'd tone up, making me look as if I'd lost more weight than I actually had. I understood the logic, but – really? It would involve parading my unfit body for all to see. The idea of being sweaty, red-faced and panting with my hair sticking up like a witch, big rolls of fat on my belly and bum shaking with every step ... no thanks.

The thing that made me change my mind about exercise was through rethinking the whole thing. Exercise didn't have to me into going to the gym, it could mean dancing, walking, gentle swimming, a game of gentle tennis ... it didn't have to mean humiliation, it could be fun, and it would help.

So I started walking.

The nice thing about walking your way to fitness is that you can start very gently and build up ... either by going faster or further as you progress. I started to set myself goals ... could I get to the end of the park in 10 minutes. Then could I get to the end of the park and back in 15 minutes. It became a challenge to beat the record I was setting myself. Playing music while I did it meant it was actually quite an uplifting experience, and it made me feel better getting more fresh air and being out and about more than I had been.

I'd always justified to myself that I wouldn't exercise because it was so painful, and also because everything I read said that it was much easier to lose weight through diet than through exercise. Even when I looked at all the research that had been done ... googling how much weight you could expect to lose with exercise, all the research was showing there was hardly any weight loss with exercise alone.

But what I found when I did it was that there were lots of benefits – it's motivating, because when you exercise as well as diet, you see changes quicker because you tone up, so it inspires you to lose more weight.

Also, remember that exercise, even if it doesn't result in direct weight loss, has a hugely beneficial impact on the body and a massive psychological impact. If I'd made the effort to get up in the morning and walk for half an hour before work, the last thing I wanted to do was eat a fatty breakfast and undo all the good when I got back.

In terms of the physical impact of exercise, most of the effects are well known...good for your heart, your bones, your muscles and your lungs. I discovered that there's also an added benefit for people like me who have yo-yo dieted so much that their metabolism is thrown completely out of sync. My doctor said that exercise can help fix a metabolism that is wrecked by yo-yo dieting. If you don't exercise your metabolism slows down, if you start moving again it will start to change and start to become better. If you've ever been obese, your metabolism will have suffered. One of the best things you can do to get your metabolism is back on track as possible is to start moving ... any gentle exercise at all will really help. It did for me.

A note from Bernie: 70% of the people who contacted me with their weight loss tips for this book said that they had done some form of physical activity as part of their weight-loss campaign. Even if it was just going for a gentle stroll a couple of times a week ... people found it helped to include activity of some sort into their lives.

SECTON FIVE

Making it a habit

CREATING HABITS

All these things are great to do, they are simple and they really don't take long at all, but you have to do them regularly to make a difference. We're all familiar with the way things work - you get into a routine and start developing healthy ways, the weight starts to come off, then you have a bad night and it all collapses, you eat badly, your head goes and suddenly all the weight goes back on, leaving you feeling hopeless as well as overweight.

You can only create new habits by changing your attitude to food and not using it as a crutch. While you're relying on food to get you through tough times, your ability to succeed is limited by events out of your control. One day something difficult happens to make you feel bad and you're at the chocolate biscuits.

You can lose weight, and you can feel really great about yourself, but only if you let yourself believe that it's JUST FOOD, and will not help if your marriage breaks up, your cleaner runs off with the family silver or you lose your job. Food can't help with those things.

You need to create new habits...this is how some readers did it:

Sarah's tip:

I broke my bad habits & created new ones

Hi, my name is Sarah, I'm 68-years-old and I have lost 50lbs. I went from 196lbs to 146lbs. I did it by sensible eating, and I think the reason I was able to lose weight when so many other people fail, is because I changed my behaviour around food by breaking my lifetime habits.

My story:
I'm so glad I've been asked to share my weight loss tips with you because I have lost 50lbs and I did it by breaking all my bad habits. I think the key to losing weight is to understand what your habits are ... what you do regularly has made you the weight you are. If you don't like that weight - break those habits.

For example, I found myself drinking loads of cups of tea at work, and every time I went to the kettle to make a cup of tea there'd be biscuits there. I'd have a biscuit while the kettle was boiling, make a cup of tea and take it back to my desk with another biscuit. I did that every time. That's around 200 calories every time I made a cup of tea. It was definitely a habit. I wasn't having a biscuit because I was hungry, but because they were there, and it was a nice thing to do while the kettle was boiling.

What I learnt when I started to think about my habit of getting up to have cups of tea all the time was that half the reason I was standing up from my desk was because I felt I needed a break, and to talk to people. It was the same at lunchtime, rather than taking healthy lunch from home, I'd always go to the cafe over the road, because that way I'd meet people and talk to them and get some fresh air. My job is very solitary - I'm a researcher in a library.

So what I decided to do was to accept that what I wanted was interaction with people, and give myself a short break every couple of hours to wander out, get some fresh air and talk to other researchers, then come back to my desk. I didn't need tea and I didn't need the biscuits and I didn't need the calorific sandwiches at lunch time. That was all just habit. Habits can be broken as soon as you identify them.

Do you have a habit of having a glass of wine every night after work? Do you convince yourself that now the bottle's open you might as well have another one? I certainly used to. It's all just habit and it's hundreds and hundreds and thousands of calories you're taking in, just because of bad habits.

It's not the body or your metabolism that's making you overweight or obese – it's your brain. That's really clear to me now, after losing weight that I had been trying to lose for half my life.

It's poor decisions that make you gain weight. Good decisions will allow you to lose it. If you're overweight, you might have been making bad decisions for a while, and the problem is that over time, the poor decisions lead to significant changes in how the brain behaves. Years of any kind of behavior pattern creates habits that take some breaking. The good news is that the brain can "fix" itself once new habits are formed.

You need to rewire your brain. The way to do this is to work out what bad habits you have around food…biscuits with tea, a glass of wine with dinner, extras, pudding, eating crisps. Keep a note of what you're eating during a week and spot patterns. Try and identify just two habits to change and change them. Work out why you're always eating a chocolate bar on the train on the way home. Is it because you're hungry? If so, have something healthier, if it's not because you're hungry – why? Tiredness, boredom, or just buying one out of habit. You need to understand yourself if you're going to lose weight – work out why you're sabotaging yourself. Once you know why you're always doing something, you can set about trying to change it…make new healthy habits and finally shift that weight.

Philippa's tip:
I became accountable

Hi, my name is Philippa. I'm 53-years-old and I have lost 44lbs. I went from 210lbs to 166lbs. I did it by making myself accountable. I decided to take weight loss seriously…treated it like a business.

My story:

My tip might sound a bit odd at first – be accountable. To whom? It's only you responsible for your weight. But the gist of my tip for you, as someone who's lost a hell of a lot of weight, and kept it off (for two years now) is to be accountable to yourself. Be organised, plan properly, treat the process like an important business campaign because in many ways it's much more important than that...this is your God damned health we're talking about here...take it seriously!

So, I decided to become accountable.... I decided to weigh myself every Monday at the same time, and keep my weight loss results on a chart next to my desk. Then I made sure I kept a food diary, listing everything I had eaten or drunk that day. I know you read a lot of diet instructions which say that you should keep a food diary, and I'd always dismissed it before, I would definitely, definitely advise doing it because it does help you see what you're eating, and where you could make little cutbacks to help lose weight.

If you make yourself accountable, and keep proper records of everything, it's really motivating when you do well. Also, when you don't do well, you can see exactly where the problems are rising (maybe in that week where you drank too much wine you didn't lose weight, so it reminds you to cut back on the booze). If you haven't kept a record of everything, you don't know how you're doing, and it's very hard to improve.

I know some people aren't naturally planners, or organisers, but even if you're not, if you can bear it you will find you get much better results if you plan carefully, monitor carefully, and record all your results. That's certainly what I found, and if you look at companies like Weight Watchers and the Cambridge diet and all those other formal diets, one of the main things they do is weigh you and give you feedback on your weight and measurements all the time. Even if you do a weight loss program in a gym, they weigh you and measure you at the beginning and give your updates as to how your plan is going. They do this because they know that if you get feedback it helps motivate you. If you're doing it yourself, like I was, you need to provide your own motivation, so you need to get yourself organised and make yourself accountable.

These are the ways I suggest you do it ... this is certainly the way I lost weight:

- Keep a food diary of everything you eat, be as honest as you possibly can, and update it regularly. No one will see this but you, but it does help you realise how you're making slipups along the way, or even to give you something to congratulate yourself on when you have a particularly good day.

- Chart your measurements and weight as the weight starts to come off. Either weigh yourself once a week or once every two weeks - it's up to you, but make sure you keep a record of what's going on.

- Get organised at home. I've found with my diet that the times I wasn't able to keep to it was when I hadn't organised myself properly. I think you have to plan your meals in advance so you know what to buy, so you've always got good food in the house. There's nothing more likely to make you eat badly than a situation where the only food in your house is pizza and crisps. Make sure this doesn't happen by being organised and planning meals in advance.

- Plan to do some exercise ... it's very easy not to do any because you're too busy. I think you have to prioritize it. You never don't eat because you're too busy, you do the things are important. I've found it really worked for me when I prioritized exercise. When I say exercise, sometimes this was going for a swim after work, other times it was just getting off the bus earlier and walking, or walking up the stairs ... just making sure I planned something into the day that counted as exercise.

- Reward yourself. The point of being accountable is that you can praise yourself as well as criticise yourself!

- Be clear about the times you allow yourself to eat. Before I went on my diet I found myself eating quite a lot late at night. I'd come back from work by about six, sort out the kids, get changed into something comfortable pour myself a glass of wine and relax then I was at my most dangerous ... crisps and dips, another glass of wine, cheese sandwich ... Now I have a rule that I must not eat after 6.30 PM unless I'm going out to dinner. So, I come back from work, prepare healthy meal for myself and my kids straight away, then I don't eat again that evening. It's really worked for me, and if I get hungry, I just drink loads and loads of water. Sparkling water is particularly filling.

Some other tips from my readers:

Mike's tip:
   I learnt from McDonalds.

Hi, my name is Mike. I'm 19-years-old and I have lost 50lbs. I went from 270lbs to 220lbs and I did it by realizing what fast food restaurants did to make you eat a lot, and I did the opposite. I'm fairly sure that my diet tip will be the most ridiculous one in this research... it's all about fooling yourself into eating less, eating less frequently, and eating more healthily by taking advice from McDonald's, Burger King, Wimpey, Wendy's and all other fast food outlets.

My story:

I was a junk food addict...eating fast food all the time. I was aware that I'd go into McDonalds and have a burger and fries and immediately want another one, but I thought that was just me being greedy. Then I saw an interesting article about how fast food outlets encourage you to spend more money. They obviously do this by trying to get you to eat more, and eat faster. It struck me that if I tried to do the opposite of what fast food restaurants do, then I would be encouraging myself to eat less and eat more slowly.
   So... here are the lessons from McDonald's that can help you lose weight:
   1.)   In McDonald's they don't have plates -- they put your food onto trays. The reason they do this is to make the food look quite small on the tray, so you don't feel as if you're eating very much. This encourages you to feel as if you can eat much more. So, the first thing I did was serve my food on the smallest plates I had in the

house. I'd just give myself a portion that could fit onto a small plates, and if I was still hungry I'd have a little bit more. Apparently this genuinely does work to make you eat less, because when a plate is full it sends messages to your brain that there's a lot of it, so your brain sends a message out that you are full much sooner than it would.

2.) In McDonald's they put food flat onto the tray, this is because when food is piled up it makes you feel as if you're eating more, so when you serve yourself at home put your food into a tall pile and it makes it look as if you've got a lot more of it (I know this sounds odd, but it's true!)

3.) McDonald's restaurants are deliberately unatmospheric; they don't want you to linger in there when you're not eating. You are not encouraged to stay for a coffee afterwards. The music they play is tinny, not conducive to sitting around for a long time while you eat. This is what makes you eat more quickly. So I started making an effort to lay the table properly, sit down with a nice atmosphere, and relish my food at home, instead of rushing it. I certainly think that if you take more time with your food, you feel yourself getting full-up more quickly, and don't reach for seconds.

4.) In McDonald's the lights are very bright, this is another way of making you eat faster. That's why lovely, expensive restaurants have candlelight.

5.) The colours ... the colours red and yellow are designed to make you want to eat, that's why McDonald's uses them. Apparently, blue is the colour that least makes you want to eat. So, next time you go to buy any new crockery, go for small plates and plates that are either blue, or white with a blue pattern (again -- the colours that you would associate with a smart restaurant).

I know this may sound like a silly tip, but I'm being honest. It was when I stopped rushing my food, ate slowly, and didn't behave like a teenager in a McDonald's restaurant that I started to really move the weight. I've actually lost 50lbs, so I desperately needed to lose weight. It was the little tricks that helped me. I wish you lots and lots of luck in your efforts to lose weight. Be kind to yourself, treat yourself nicely, and whatever you do don't behave like a starving teenager in a McDonald's restaurant.

Jen's story:
   Tapping

Hi, my name is Jen. I'm 53-years-old and I have lost 40lbs. I went from 180lbs to 140lbs and I did it by learning the art of tapping. I find it calms me down, gives me breathing space and has stopped my frenetic eating.

My story:

OK, before we start, I should tell you that this is nothing to do with tap dancing. When I told my husband that I was going to try tapping to lose weight, he said straight away "well don't do it in here, we have wooden floors, the guys in the apartment downstairs will be horrified." But it's nothing to do with dance. Tapping is a way of relaxing yourself, getting control of yourself, and getting rid of urges and this all happens by tapping yourself with your fingers.

I'm well aware of how ridiculous this all sounds, but by tapping certain parts of your face arms and shoulders that have been identified as linked to urges, you do manage to get control over yourself, and stop eating so much. At least I did.

My tip is to try tapping – what have you got to lose? It definitely, definitely worked for me. I'm 53 now, and when I was 48 I'd almost given up hope of ever losing weight. I saw tapping mentioned in a newspaper article, and gave it a go. I bought a book, but I don't think you even need to do that, you just need to know where to tap, and when to do it, and if you're anything like me it will make all the difference in the world. I don't know how or why – I don't understand any of the science behind it (though apparently there's lots of science behind it), all I know is that the theory is that it helps bridge the gap between your body and your mind, allowing you to do a small physical movement that sends a strong signal to the brain.

So, below I've listed exactly what I did to lose weight through tapping. It's just a few stages, but it is worth going through these stages properly for you to have the maximum benefit.

Stage One

The hardest thing about losing weight through tapping is that you have to work out what is making you eat in the first place. So you will have to spend a bit of time thinking about yourself, and what is making you behave the way you are. If you always have something to eat after a row with your kids, a row with the boss, or a difficult commute into work - these are the things that you are going to be tapping to get rid of. You can tap directly to get rid of your desire to eat all the time, or your anger that you've put on so much weight, but I personally started doing this, then the more I read about it, realise that the more specific the thing you are tapping for, the greater the results.

I realised that I was reaching out for food when I got off the train after my really stressful commute to work every morning. By tapping away the stress I felt, I stopped myself eating the half a packet of biscuits, crisps and cakes that I had once consumed.

This worked for me, because I had established before starting tapping that it was my stressful commute that was causing me the most emotional pressure, and most likely lead me to emotional eating. I recommend that you do this first before starting the tapping.

Stage Two

Next, you need to work out how much stress you're feeling in certain circumstances – do this simply by thinking about yourself in a situation…dealing with your boss, when the baby is crying, when you're trying to sort out your finances ... whatever it is, write a score down for how angry, cross or upset it makes you feel. If you don't feel anything at all about that particular scenario, give it a zero. This bit is all about gut instinct, so don't think about it for too long -- just write down whatever you're feeling, and give it a score.

Stage Three

You need to create a statement which encompasses how you are feeling (ie: stressed about the commute), but in the statement you say that you won't let the feeling control you.

So, my statement was: 'I acknowledge that I feel stressed and angry when I drive into work, I accept how I feel and I am OK.'

The one I did specifically mentioning weight loss was: "Even though I am angry that I have put on three stone, I accept who I am, and I'm OK.'

One friend I spoke to said she didn't feel 'angry' at putting on weight, but very, very upset, so she changed the word 'angry' for 'upset' – you need to get this word right, because it's that emotion that we're trying to banish.

Stage four

This is where you get tapping:

There are 10 stages – do each of these while saying your statement three times in each phase.

1. Tap with two fingers from one hand on the fleshy part of the hand below the little finger on the other hand, while saying your statement three times.

2. Tap inside the eyebrow, while saying your statement three times.

3. Tap the outer edge of the eye, while saying your statement three times.

4. Tap under your eye, at the lower edge of the eye socket, while saying your statement three times.

5. Tap under your nose, while saying your statement three times.

6. Tap under your chin, while saying your statement three times.

7. Tap your collarbone, while saying your statement three times.

8. Tap your armpit, while saying your statement three times.

9. Tap the top of your head, while saying your statement three times.

Now ask yourself whether you feel better about the issues that led you to over eat. Rate yourself again and see whether your number has dropped…if it has – brilliant! Repeat that every day. Eventually you can move to a more positive statement: 'I'm happy that I no longer eat all the time and feel I have control over myself'.

I know this might not work for everyone, and I know how daft it sounds, but it worked brilliantly for me.

So...there you have it. Some tips from me and from my readers who have got in touch. If you want to share any tips with me, any funny stories or observations, please do, and we'll include them in new editions of this book.

To end this book, I'd just like to repeat something that I wrote at the beginning:

If you are overweight it's not because you're a bad person, you didn't kill anyone, you didn't steal anything, or hit anyone, or do anything criminal. You just ate too much because you felt low, or got into a habit of eating while bored. That's not a crime. Most importantly, it can be changed.

If you eat a bag of chips tonight or eight packet of biscuits, the world won't end, just shrug it off, wake up tomorrow and try to go for a 10 minute walk and have a glass of water. No one ever lost weight by beating themselves up and feeling bad.

Now – there follows one of my novels 'Adorable Fat Girl goes to weight loss camp'. I hope you enjoy it.

Bernie x

ADORABLE FAT GIRL GOES TO WEIGHT LOSS CAMP

NOTHING BUT CARROTS

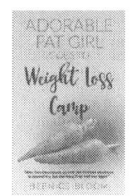

I was all curled up on mum's sofa, clutching a sweet cup of tea and feeling its warmth against the palms of my hands, as rain hammered against the windows. It had been pouring all day and was now coming down so hard that you could hear it hitting the conservatory roof like gunfire. Darkness had started to descend. It was only 7pm for God's sake. Outside it looked like the end of the world.

"I should go home soon," I said. "But this rain is just awful. I can't face going out in it."

"No, don't be ridiculous. You can't go anywhere til it stops. Just relax and enjoy your tea. Stay for something to eat and your dad will run you back later."

"Thanks mum," I said, snuggling further down into the sofa and feeling all safe and secure. The theme tune for the One Show came on and I don't think I'd ever felt cosier in my life. I clutched my mug between my hands and blew onto the scalding liquid, watching the steam fly up onto my face, warming my nose. It was like I was giving myself a mini steam facial.

"How are things going then?" asked mum, eying me with confusion as I tried to get the steam to hit my chin where I'm particularly prone to blackheads. "What on earth are you trying to do with that mug?"

"Nothing," I said, continuing to hold the mug in position. You'd pay £40 for this sort of treatment at the beauticians.

"You seem a bit out of sorts. Is everything OK with you and Ted?"

I shrugged, not because things weren't going well with my boyfriend, but because I now had my chin right over the top of the mug and didn't want to move.

"For the love of God, are you having some sort of breakdown over there? Or are you trying to drink your tea through your chin?"

"Neither," I said, reluctantly putting down the mug. "I was just warming up my chin."

"Warming up your chin?"

"Yes. My chin was cold, that's all." I crossed my arms over my chest and turned to watch the television. They had just started a segment about window boxes.

"You and Ted aren't getting on well, are you?" she said, her voice full of anxiety. "He's such a lovely man, it would be a shame if you messed this up."

"Things are fine," I replied, turning my attention back to the planting taking place in the BBC studio. "He works long hours and I've been away a lot recently, so we haven't seen all that much of one another, but everything's just fine."

"Oh," she said. "Doesn't sound like things are 'just fine' if you never see him. And 'fine' is such an odd word to use. I thought you two were in love."

"We are. Honestly, mum, we're both doing really well and the relationship's great, I just want to see what they do with these primroses."

"OK," she said, taking a large gulp of tea, but she looked far from OK. She clearly wanted to talk but I genuinely wanted to see what they would put next to the primroses. I work in a gardening and DIY store, and I have been charged with sorting out all the window boxes next week. I needed tips from Alan Titchmarsh.

Mum fell into a respectful silence while the colourful, floral creations took shape. Then the programme moved onto Phil Tufnell talking about the plight of urban foxes. Mum seized her moment and grabbed the remote control, hitting the pause button and leaving poor Phil frozen on the screen. I knew what was coming.

"Come on then," she said. "Tell me what the trouble is."

"There's no trouble. Honestly, mum. Ted and I are very happy."

"But there's no talk of you moving in together? No talk of wedding bells?"

"No talk like that at all, mum. But we're happy so stop worrying."

"I do worry, I can't help it," she said. "You were always so sad and out of sorts until Ted came along...he's transformed you. He's a lovely man. I'd hate to see things going wrong."

"They won't. Everything's fine. Now can we talk about something else, or I'll put the foxes back on."

"OK. You can talk to me anytime you want, if you're worried about anything."

"I know," I said. "And I will if I'm worried about anything." Although the one thing I'm absolutely sure of is that my mother would be the last person on the planet I'd talk to if I was having problems with my relationship.

"What are you up to, then?" she asked. "Any exciting trips planned?"

"Well, Ted and I are talking about going to America in the summer. He's looking at what sort of holiday we could do. I fancy a road trip - you know - take in a lot of places all in one visit. Route 66 and all that."

"I thought you were going somewhere else as well," said mum. "Like a health place or something?"

"Yes, I'm off on a weight loss retreat in Portugal next week. I told you all about that."

"A weight loss retreat. That's right," she mused, offering me a chocolate biscuit. I took one, of course. Always better to discuss the merits of weight loss retreats while dunking heavily-coated chocolate hobnobs into devilishly sweet tea.

"All they'll give you to eat at weight loss retreats is carrots. You do know that, don't you?"

3

"I'm sure that's not ALL we'll be given," I replied. "I'm sure there'll be other food."

"Nope...carrot juice, carrots in salads and carrots on their own - carrots lying on the plate in front of you, taunting you with their orangeness. By the end of the week you'll be having nightmares about carrots taking over the country. Just talk to Aunty Susan, she went on a Fat Camp when she was 20, before her wedding, and she was definitely a light orangey colour when she came home. Take a look at the wedding photos. Looks like Donald Trump, she does."

"She does not. I've seen her wedding photos, she looks lovely in them."

"Lovely, yes, but apricot coloured. I mean, apricot's a nice colour for a blouse or a summer skirt, but not for your face. In the wedding photos she looked like she's been living too close to a nuclear plant or been bathing in cheesy wotsits or something."

"Well, even if it was all about carrots back then, it's not now. Also, it's definitely not called 'Fat Camp'. You're talking about something from the 1950s, it's all different today. I'm going on a weight loss retreat and will have healthy food, fresh air and exercise and I'll come back energised and looking a lot like Jennifer Lawrence. It will be brilliant."

"Do you have to write about it again on that blog thing?"

"Yep," I said. "Another free trip."

I've got myself a nice little gig writing for my friend Dawn's blog. It's called 'Two Fat Ladies' and because I'm rather well-upholstered she invites me to help her review various holidays, The trouble is - things always go wrong.

This is the third trip I've managed to wangle myself onto. I've been on safari (got stuck up a tree in my knickers and it all ended up on webcam - disaster!) and went on a cruise (befriended a 90-year-old man and a flamboyant dancer and managed to miss the ship and bump into an ex-boyfriend - disaster!).

I'm hoping that this one will be straightforward and I'll come back looking thin and lovely without having created any colossal dramas along the way.

"Well I hope you're right. I hope that fat camps have changed since your Aunty Susan went," said mum, with a raise of her eyebrows. A smile played upon her lips and a look of furtive shame crept across her features. "It was funny though, hearing all the stories. I remember Susan telling me about when she escaped and went running to the pub with one of the other women, and the pub landlord guessed what they'd done and called the Fat Camp owner who sent out two guys to collect them and bring them back. They were even frisked back at Fat Club and two packets of pork scratchings were found in your Aunty Susan's knickers. Don't tell her I told you that though, will you? We called her piggy pants for ages afterwards...don't tell her I told you that either."

I smiled as I thought about my sensible aunty having pub snacks hidden in her girdle.

"I won't be like that," I said. "I want to go and do it properly and lose loads of weight so I can start on a proper health and fitness drive and really get down to a healthy, sensible weight."

"Good girl," said mum. "You won't want another one of these, then."

Mum took a hob nob and bit into it slowly, while I flicked through the weight loss camp brochure.

"Most people lose 7lbs on the holiday," I read out.

"That'll be the carrots," she replied through a mouth full of biscuit. I ignored her and carried on reading.

"If you join the running group you can expect to dramatically increase the speed and distance you can run."

"Yep, everyone running away from carrots," she said.

"There's no mention of bloody carrots in the brochure. They talk about healthy, organic food that will fill you up and give you the strength you need to exercise while allowing you to shed all the weight you want."

"The carrots are a secret."

"For the love of God, mum. Shut up about the carrots."

. . .

A week later, Aunty Susan came over for lunch with Uncle Mark and I knew the subject of my pending Weight Loss holiday would be raised. Mum was dying to have her theories about the holiday confirmed.

"I was telling Mary about the Fat Camp that you went on before your wedding, Sue," she said.

"Oh God!" said Aunty Susan, dropping her cutlery so it clattered on her plate. "That was terrible. Do you remember? Me and that other lady tried to escape but they came and caught us."

"I never knew about that," said Mark. "Where did you try to escape to?"

"To the pub and the fish and chip shop," replied Susan. "They caught us in the pub, I think, before we'd even had the chance to get to the fish and chip shop."

"Why would you try to escape?" Mark asked. "I thought you liked going to spas and things like that."

I braced myself.

"I love spas, but this place was dreadful…they made us exercise from 5am til 8pm, and fed us nothing but carrots."

"You see," said mum, turning around to face me with a look of triumph on her face. "What did I tell you? Nothing but carrots."

MUM ON TOUR

While mum sat and explained to Aunty Susan how she'd been warning me about the carrots, my phone rang. Dawn's number appeared on the screen, so I excused myself and wandered into the kitchen.

"Hi Flairy, zits fawn," said Dawn's familiar voice.

"Sorry? I couldn't understand a word of that."

I could hear mum and Aunty Susan laughing uproariously as they were telling Uncle Mark all about the Fat Camp she'd been on. I noticed that they didn't mention her hiding pork scratchings in her knickers though. I must make sure to mention that.

"It's Fawn," said the voice on the phone.

"Fawn?"

"No, Dawn. Sorry - I've got a mouthful of food."

"Not carrots, I hope."

"No, of course not. I'm eating cake. Why would you think I'd be eating carrots?"

"Just something my mum was saying earlier about everyone at weight loss Camp eating nothing but carrots."

"Well, your mum will be able to find out for herself if she wants," said Dawn.

"What do you mean?"

"I mean she will literally be able to find out for herself. The organisers of the weight loss camp say you can take your mum with you because they are keen to advertise a Mother's' Day special that they are running next month. They thought that would make an interesting angle for the blog and I agree with them to be honest. You know 'weight loss camp with my mum'. I think it could be really funny for readers."

I was silent. I wasn't expecting this at all.

"Mary, are you still there?" asked Dawn.

"Yes, still here, but shocked into silence," I said. "I can't take my mum with me."

"Come on, it would make great copy. Can you imagine it...you're really witty, Mary, and have got yourself a great following already. Weight watching with your mum will add a whole new dimension to that. Readers will love it. Readers will think it's really funny as they hear all about the two of you."

"Yeah, funny for readers, but hell on earth for me."

"I'm sure your mum is lovely."

"She is," I said, as mum walked past me to get more drink. She pulled out a fresh bottle of sherry and I realised they were in for a long night...when she and Aunty Susan get cracking on the sherry there's no stopping them: they'll be dancing to Elvis and Buddy Holly in no time. "But mum's not fat. I can't take my mum on a weight loss camp if she doesn't need to lose weight, that would be crazy."

"Ooooooo..." said mum, stopping in the doorway with her bottle of sherry and spinning round to face me. "Yes, you can take me to weight loss camp with you. I definitely need to lose a few pounds," she said. "Everyone over the age of 60 needs to lose weight. I used to be so slim and elegant. Not anymore though. Take me with you, Mary, we'd have such fun."

"Let me talk this through with her and I'll come back to you" I said to Dawn, as I ended the call and followed mum into the sitting room. Mum was in there flexing her muscles at Aunty Susan. She had rolled up the short sleeves of her silk top and was displaying arms with the merest hint of flabby skin hanging beneath them. This was supposed to indicate how overweight she was.

"Isn't it awful," she was saying to Aunty Susan, as she gently nudged her arm and shook her head as it rippled. "However slim you keep yourself, you can't help it when you get older."

"I wouldn't worry, mum, I've got more loose flesh than that on my ankles," I said.

"So, am I coming?"

"I don't think it will be your sort of thing," I tried. "I mean - when have you ever shown any interest in health and fitness?"

"Excuse me, Madam, but when have you?" asked mum.

I nodded at her. She had a point. Though, in my defence, I do talk a lot about getting fit...I just don't do anything about it. Does it count if you talk about it endlessly?

"I took up yoga," I said, remembering my weekend retreat a while ago. "I wore nothing but bloody Lycra for days."

"Well, that's true," said mum. "But how much yoga did you actually do? It sounds to me like you spent most of the time falling over and ogling men in tight shorts."

Again, she wasn't wrong.

"I think it would be lovely if we went to the weight loss camp together. I mean, I understand if you say you don't want me to go with you, but I'd really like to."

"Ah, go on Mary, take her," said Aunty Susan. "She'll be very well-behaved."

Oh God, why was this so hard?

"But remember what you said about the carrots," I said. "You wouldn't want to have to eat carrots for every meal, would you?"

"I wouldn't mind," said mum. "I wouldn't mind what I ate as long as I was with you."

Bugger, bugger, bugger. What could I possibly say to that?

"Of course I'd like you to come, mum," I told her, with a heavy heart. I'd imagined myself frolicking on the beach with handsome instructors and flirting outrageously with the tennis coaches before sneaking out for late night glasses of wine with the other guests, not to mention the snacks I was planning to take. Now it looked like it was going to be all fitness classes and games of Scrabble.

"Ooo, what fun," mum said. "Don't worry about a thing now, Mary. I'll be there to keep you on the straight and narrow and out of trouble."

"That's what I'm worried about," I said.

It was five days to go before the weight loss retreat and I was trying so hard to be good. I didn't want to look like a pot-bellied pig in my bikini. Going with mum added a whole new level of stress to the trip; she was so lovely and slim - I didn't want everyone to be looking at us both and wondering why on earth I was so huge when she was so tiny. I thought that at least if I lay off the booze and cut back on the snacks I'd look a bit better…just a bit.

"I'm not going to drink tonight," I said to Ted, refusing a glass, and taking a sip of his wine when his back was turned. "I'm going to be good."

"Um…" said Ted, having seen me stealing his glass out of the corner of his eye. "For someone who's not going to drink tonight you seem to be drinking a hell of a lot of my wine."

"Everyone knows that calories taken off someone else's plate or from someone else's glass don't count," I advised.

"Right," said Ted, looking highly dubious.

"It's a flawless plan, to be fair," I said, taking another large sip from his glass.

"Just have a glass of wine if you want glass of wine, woman." he said. "You're not going to get any fatter drinking your own glass instead of my glass."

God love him; does he know nothing?

"By the way, what are you doing tomorrow? Do you fancy coming to the football with me?" he said. "There's a group of us going, it will be a laugh."

"I'd rather sit at home and stick pins in my eyes - why would I want to go to the football?"

"All the other girlfriends go," he said in whiny voice. "They talk among themselves, you don't have to watch the football...just come along and have a beer and mix with everyone."

"Next time," I said. "I'm going holiday shopping with mum tomorrow to get supplies for our trip." Heaven help me; I'm not sure which is the worse day out - football with Ted and his lager lout friends or clothes shopping with mum.

"Blimey, are you sure you wouldn't rather come to the football?"

"I have to go with her," I said. "If I don't it will be an utter disaster. Yesterday she was talking about buying a jazzy pink headband and ankle warmers to wear to the fitness classes. If I don't take her in hand she'll look like Jane Fonda's grandmother. I need to go with her to make sure she doesn't lose her mind in Sports Direct."

"OK, well - rather you than me - if you change your mind, come down to the football - you know where we'll be."

"I will," I said.

The next day I woke with a heavy heart at the thought of the delights ahead of me. My mum is lovely, she really is, and I'm sure your mum is too, but would you want to go on holiday with her? Honestly? And would you want to go shopping for fitness wear with her in advance of the holiday? You don't need to answer that; we all know the answer.

I caught the bus over to mum's house in Esher first thing in the morning and picked her up, then the two of us went on the bus into Kingston. She was so chirpy and thrilled at the idea of going shopping with me that I felt really bad for all the things I'd been thinking. I decided to be positive and upbeat and make this whole experience something that mum would love.

"Where shall we go first?" asked mum. Her cheeks were all flushed and she looked really excited that we were out on a shopping trip. I swear, you'd think I never went anywhere with her, or that she had never been shopping before. "I suppose you'll want to go to Topshop or Zara - or some of those other young person's shops, won't you?" she said. "I'll come with you, but will need to get my clothes somewhere a little more age-appropriate."

I didn't want to tell mum that the clothes in Topshop hadn't fitted me since puberty, and I hadn't been in Zara since I got stuck in a dress there and ended up ripping it in an effort to get it off.

"I was thinking about the department stores - John Lewis and Bentalls, and maybe Marks and Spencer," I said. I knew they were the most likely shops to stock a swimming costume that was big enough for me. I also needed a cover-all kaftan so I didn't scare the locals and a summery dress in case there was a cocktail party one evening. "Do those shops sound OK?"

"Yes, very nice," she said, looking delighted with my suggestions. "And we don't have to worry about paying for lunch because I've bought sandwiches with me." She opened her bag to reveal cling film wrapped bread at the bottom, and a flask."

"That's soup in there. It's Heinz so it should be nice. And I've got boiled eggs for us to have with the sandwiches. They're here, somewhere."

"Great," I said, as mum rummaged around on her egg hunt. "We'll go to the park after shopping for a picnic."

Mum brightened further at the thought of that.

We decided to go to Sports Direct first, mainly because we walked right past it when we got off the bus, but also because mum wanted trainers and dad had persuaded her that the only decent place to buy trainers was a sports shop.

"Your father says that I mustn't buy cheap ones from a supermarket, I've got to buy proper ones from a sports shop or I'll slip and break my hip or something."

"OK," I said, and in we went. Mum tried on a succession of shoes and as she skipped around the shop, testing them out, I thought how youthful she looked - she was very young-looking for her age and didn't have an ounce of fat on her.

"I think I'll take these pink ones," she said, with a girlish smile. "Shall I get you some too?"

"I'd look ridiculous in them," I said. "I only wear black trainers."

"Well, I think you should get some brightly coloured ones. You'd look lovely in these."

"No mum, honestly, it's really kind of you, but last time I wore pink I look like Tinky Winky so I've stopped all bright colours until I lose weight."

"Let me buy you something," said mum. "Choose whatever you fancy as a treat from me."

I didn't want to buy anything in the sports shop. Nothing looks more ridiculous than a woman who's clearly not done a moment's exercise since the 1990s, all dressed up in brand new exercise gear, especially if the gear is three sizes too small.... which it would have been if I'd attempted to buy something in there.

After the shoe shopping, we went upstairs and mum bought some very lovely, deeply-flattering Lycra sportswear. I can't tell you how annoying it is when your mum looks better in clothes than you do. I could have hit her as she emerged from the changing rooms saying: "Could you get one of these for me in a size 10, Mary? This one's far too big for me."

As I watched her, I kept thinking 'why am I fat, and she's not?' I mean - how does the whole overeating thing work? Surely, you'd think that I would be fat because my mum is fat, and she over fed me from a young age, or gave me a negative relationship with food, or something. But it doesn't seem to work like that - I seem to be unable to stop eating and unable to stop thinking about eating, whereas mum just eats when she's hungry.

Our relationships with food are so different. It's like food means a different thing in both our lives - to me it's a joyous thing hovering on the horizon, never quite out of sight, always alluring and always exciting. When there's food in the room it's like I become a person possessed...I can't relax til it's all eaten, and when I eat it it's like I can't get enough of it, like there's no amount of food that's ever going to satisfy me, ever going to fill me up and allow me to relax. I just wish I didn't have to eat ever again. I wish eating wasn't part of life.

"Right," said mum, returning to me with all her purchases packed away in a carrier bag. "Let's go and have a picnic in the park, shall we?"

"Oooh yes," I said, trotting along beside her, my maudlin mood lifted a little by the thought of food (see what I mean? It's insane).

"Shall we walk down to the grassy bank that we went past on the bus a little earlier? It seemed nice there, didn't it?"

"Or we could go just here," I said, indicating a small park that was not as nice as the spot that mum was talking about, but was nearer, meaning we could eat sooner and I wouldn't have to walk for ages.

"I thought the spot by the river was nicer?"

"No - the ducks and geese come there and they're really vicious," I said. "This will be much better." I threw down my coat as a makeshift blanket before mum could attempt to make me change my mind.

"OK," she said, and started unloading the picnic. I felt instantly bad for making her sit there. I'm just horrible when there's food around.

"We can go back to the river if you like," I said.

"No, said mum, opening a very small packet of sandwiches. "Don't worry. This is just perfect."

SOLDIERING ALONG

The flight left on a Monday, while Ted was at work, so the task of taking two women and bags full of leisurewear to the airport fell to dad.

"Now have you both definitely got everything," he said, once we were in the car with our luggage in the boot. "Check now, before we leave."

We both rummaged through our respective handbags and said we were OK. We had our passports with us and that's all that mattered.

"You don't need tickets?" asked dad.

"Err no - it's all magic now," I said. "They are e-tickets - on my phone."

"Have you got the information about the camp and how we get there?" asked mum.

I pulled an envelope out of my bag. "All in here," I said. I hadn't opened it, but I knew it was all there. With that we were off - chugging along the motorway on our journey to Heathrow.

AFTER CHECKING in and passing through security with an alarming lack of hassle or incident, mum and I headed for the beauty counters in the duty-free shop.

I sprayed a liberal amount of Chanel No5 onto my wrists and neck and tipped way too much body lotion into my hands so that I ended up spreading it all the way up my arms to get rid of it. Mum was peering into a small mirror at the skin care counter next to me, wrinkling up her nose in disgust at the sight of herself. "You've no idea how bloody hideous it is," she said.

"How hideous what is, mum?" I replied. The lipstick she'd tried on seemed perfectly acceptable to me.

"Ageing... Waking up in the morning and discovering that your jawline has drop so far that your jowls are resting on your shoulders, and your eyes have disappeared completely – hidden behind bags, wrinkles and a forehead that's dropped four inches."

I should tell you at this stage that mum is really attractive; she is slim, elegant and always has perfect hair (You know how some people are like that... They always have the most gorgeous hair, where is mine is hit and miss – regardless of what I do with it, sometimes it looks okay and other times it looks terrible for no reason at all).

Anyway – what I'm saying is mum looks good, and she's not all that vain, so the small outburst as she peered into the mirror came as a bit of a shock.

"You look great mum, what are you talking about?"

"I'm talking about the unwanted hairs popping up on my chin, the grey roots and the beachball that has appeared where my waistline used to be. The only thing I've got in my favour is that I haven't got incontinence or piles, unlike Aunty Susan."

"Yeah, thanks mum. I really needed to know that."

"And the reason for that is because I do daily pelvic floor exercises and it makes the world of difference. You should start now. I'll show you when we get to the room. Honestly, I do them so often it's a wonder I can't get my pelvic floor up to touch the back of my throat."

"Oh God, mum."

I turned to look at the mascaras. My eyes are the only part of me that I like. I have big eyes, you see. In fact, I have big everything, but big eyes are allowed. Have you ever thought about that? I have really big feet and that's frowned upon. Having size eight feet is not ladylike. Having big thighs is not good and neither is having a big tummy. But big eyes? That's good; that's allowed. A big smile is allowed too, but not a big neck.

I need to go and live in a country where all big is beautiful and my huge arse is celebrated as much as my huge eyes. Maybe Tonga or somewhere. Isn't the King of Tonga chosen as king because he's the fattest person in the country? Christ, I'd be running the place in the blink of an eye.

I turned back to mum to find her holding her forehead up with her index fingers so that her eyebrows were raised, and she was pulling the sides of her face out with her thumbs.

"Do I look young?" she asked.

I didn't know what the right answer was. If I said "yes" that would imply that I thought she looked old normally, but if I said "No" then she'd think that even when she rearranged her features with her fingers, she still looked old.

"You look startled," I told her. "Not a good look, if you don't mind me saying. Now come on, let's go and get a drink. I want to tell you about all my plans to move to Tonga."

It was only a swift visit to the pub (mum wasn't such a fan of all day drinking as I'd hoped she'd be), then I rushed into Boots and bought more miniature toiletry items than either of us could reasonably get through in a decade, as well as stocking up on medical supplies for the flight in such quantities that we could have opened a small on-board hospital. Then it was time to board.

ON THE PLANE, I settled myself into my seat and nervously raised my hand to attract the attention of the attendant.

"Can I help you?" she asked in a loud voice.

"I'll need a seatbelt extension please," I said.

"A what?"

"A seat belt extender," I said, doing actions to mimic the putting on of a seatbelt rather than raise my voice.

"Of course, madam," she said, scurrying off to find one.

"You don't need a seatbelt extender," said mum, valiantly rushing to my defence. "You're not that fat."

I love that she's so protective, but her loyalty is verging on blindness. The seat-belt extender only just goes around me.

"Shall we have a little drink on the plane?" I suggested.

"Tea?" she said.

"Gin?" I responded.

"Are you an alcoholic?" she asked.

"What? Because I fancy a little drink on the plane on the way to holiday?"

"No, because it's a weight loss camp and only a nutcase would order alcohol on the way to it.... a nutter, or someone who loved drinking so much they couldn't help themselves. Someone with a problem, perhaps?"

"It's going to be a long five days," I muttered under my breath, as we both ordered tea. "A long, long time."

We arrived at Faro airport and I pulled the letter out of my bag to work out where we were supposed to be. I slid my finger along the seal and tore the envelope open, pulling out the pages inside.

"Let's see, it's called... 'Forces Fitness,'" I said, noticing the military-style logo at the top of the information sheet.

"Forces fitness?" said mum. "What do you mean? Like military training? Drill sergeants and press ups in the mud?"

Mum and I looked at one another.

"Forces Fitness? Shit," I said. "I thought it would be all fruit kebabs and sparkling elderflower juice. I don't fancy military fitness at all."

"It can't be," said mum. "Was there information with the letter? What does it say?"

"I didn't really look," I confessed, flicking through all the other pages in the envelope which announced that the camp was a military style fitness experience.

"Oh God...look mum."

Two men dressed in army fatigues were marching up to us, clutching clipboards. One of them was around my age and desperately handsome with chiselled features and big shoulders. He looked tough and manly but he also had long eyelashes and sea green eyes. He looked as if he could handle himself in a fight, but would also be nice to kittens and always remember your birthday. The other man was older and looked as if he would crush kittens with his bare hands and force feed them to you on your birthday. It was odd because the younger man was bigger and much stronger-looking, but somehow had a warmth about him that was lacking in his mate. The older man snarled at me.

"Names?" he said as if I was a prisoner who'd just been captured. I felt like turning around and running back through security and onto the plane and demanding that it take me right back to London. I couldn't face this week if it comprised of them shouting and calling me useless and hopeless in an effort to break me down. I'm broken enough, I need building not breaking, for God's sake.

"Didn't you hear me?" he said. "I need your names and I need your passports to be surrendered."

"OK, well I'm Mary and this is my mum," I replied, directing my comment to the handsome man. "And why do we have to 'surrender' our passports, are we being arrested or something?"

"Passports," he said.

Mum obediently rummaged in her handbag to find hers, but I wasn't interested in playing their silly games.

"I've told you our names, what are yours?"

"Staff A and Staff B," replied the man, adding: "We don't do first names."

Oh God.

"Look, we only want to lose a few pounds. Neither of us is plan-

BERNICE BLOOM

ning to invade anywhere and we have no desire to fight anyone. I just want a nice relaxing week."

"OK Mary," he said, putting his face right next to mine in quite a threatening way. "We'll see what we can do. Follow me."

Mum and I half-walked, half-skipped behind the two men who strode out in front. The only compensatory factor was that the handsome man (who I think was Staff B) had the most incredible tight bum.

I could see that mum was struggling beside me. She did a little run to keep up and moved her bag from one hand to the other. He could have offered to carry it for her. I mean - I know they're doing this whole 'tough guy' thing, but mum's not far off 70, for God's sake.

I took the bag out of mum's hand and carried it along with my own, struggling to keep up with them as they marched ahead. Then a very tall man appeared beside me. He was long and lean with round glasses and a mop of sandy blond hair

"Let me take that," he said, relieving me of mum's bag. He had a warm, friendly face and looked a little shy - not at all like the other two guys.

"Do you work for the fitness camp," I asked, wondering why he wasn't all dressed up in army fatigues.

"No. I'm a guest," he said. "I'm Simon."

Oh, I see. "I'm Mary," I said, smiling at him. He had lovely warm eyes. There was something tender and likable about him. He wasn't conventionally good looking, but had charisma. When he smiled his whole face lit up. I noticed that mum had speeded up and was talking to the fearsome-looking army guys.

"So, are you looking forward to this week?" I asked him. "To be honest, I'm terrified of what they're going to get us doing. I didn't realise it was a military fitness thing. I thought it would be Slimming World in the sunshine."

"You'll be fine," he said with a small laugh. "I mean - it's not quite Slimming World but I'm sure you'll enjoy it. I've been on one of these camps before and they're good fun once you get going. Don't worry. These guys act tough but they're good at what they do, and if you listen to them, you'll lose a lot of weight and feel great by Friday."

I smiled at him adoringly and thought how much more fun this whole holiday would be now that I had someone to chat to and flirt a little with. Not that I fancied him...he just had a nice manner, and clearly liked me, which was lovely.

"Are you very fit?" I said. "If you don't mind me asking. I'm worried that I won't be fit enough to keep up."

"Not really," said Simon. "I cycle every day but I'm not super fit so don't worry. On a camp like this you'll find that there's always someone fitter than you and someone less fit than you."

I didn't imagine they'd find someone less fit than me, but I appreciated the comment, so I smiled happily at Simon and thanked him.

"Do you mind if I ask you something?" he said, looking a little embarrassed.

"Of course," I said, fluttering my eyelashes, delighted that I'd coated them in brown owl mascara at the airport.

"I'm always blunt when it comes to seeing a lady that I'm attracted to, I don't like to hang back."

"Oh," I said, feeling my heart beating a little faster. "OK then. What did you want to ask me?"

I knew he was going to ask whether I was single. I felt excited at the prospect, but what should I say? I was tempted to lie so that I could keep the magic alive between the two of us...it would make the week so much more fun if I had someone to flirt with. But it seemed really bad of me not to mention Ted.

"What I wanted to ask you was - who's that lady who was with you earlier, the one whose bag I'm carrying? She's really attractive."

What?

"THAT'S MY MUM!" I growled.

"Oh," he said. "Is your dad on the trip?"

"No," I replied. "But my mum and dad are still together, so keep your hands off her."

"OK," he said, looking a little shocked by my outburst. "But if your mum and dad ever split up, I'd be really interested."

"Get away from me," I said, making shooing motions at him. "Go on; go away."

My bloody mother! What the hell did it say for my attractiveness if men preferred my mum? Christ, this was going to be a marvellous few days.

FOUR VILLAS IN THE SUNSHINE

We all climbed into the back of a small minibus. There was me, mum, Simon who I had completely gone off and was keen to keep as far from my mum as possible, and one of the army blokes (the handsome one). The older, angrier army guy had gone back to meet the rest of the group in his inimitable, gentle style. He arrived back a few minutes later with another couple of people: a woman called Karen and a guy called Graham.

Karen looked utterly terrified as she took her seat and looked up at the two army guys.

"They aren't as horrible as they look," I whispered to her, though I had no evidence for that - I just couldn't stand to see her looking so downcast and sad. She smiled weakly and muttered 'good', before turning to smile at mum.

"Sorry, I didn't catch your name," said Graham, so I introduced myself and mum and completely ignored Simon.

"What's your sports specialism?" said Graham.

What?

"Um. I don't really have one," I said. "I mean - I was a really good gymnast years ago, when I was young - but I wouldn't say I had a sports specialism now. Why? Are we supposed to have one?"

I looked at Staff B who was watching us with amusement from his position in the front seat. Despite the heat he had a long-sleeved shirt on and these white gloves. He must be boiling.

"No one needs any sort of specialty. We're planning to work you hard so you get the most out of the week but you won't have to do anything you don't want to. Please stop worrying."

"Does your angry-looking mate know that?" I asked. "Only he looks ready to waterboard us if we put a foot wrong."

"Don't mention waterboarding," said Staff B, suddenly getting very serious. "Never mention it. We've all been in the army, we've all experienced terrible things. Please - just don't mention it."

"OK," I said meekly, looking at mum. "Sorry."

"But in answer to your question - yes, my angry mate does know, and he's not expecting any sporting prowess either. And don't worry. His bark is worse than his bite."

"Phew," said Simon. "I don't have any particular sporting prowess. I don't know what I'd say my skills were."

"Fancying old ladies," I said under my breath, as Staff A reappeared at the side of the mini bus, looking concerned.

"I can't find her," he said.

"No, there's no one else coming," said Staff B. "We're all here. I've just checked the list. Shall we make a move?"

"No - there's someone else coming," said Staff A. "You know - the girl. I mentioned her."

"Of course," said Staff B. "Fucking hell, how could I forget. Go find her. I'll stay here." Then he turned back round to face us.

"We're just waiting for one other person to arrive," he said. "She's coming on the Manchester flight. She'll be here any minute."

I turned my attention to mum, who'd gone very quiet.

"Everything OK?" I asked.

"Yes, just feeling a bit tired now. I could do with a nap. Travelling is exhausting when you're older."

"Have a little nap now," I suggested, bundling up my jumper and her coat behind her head so she could lean back on the window. I looked up to see Simon smiling at her. He swung his head away when he saw me looking.

Minutes later Staff A emerged from the airport building with a very glamorous brunette, strikingly slim in white jeans and white t-shirt with gold high-heeled sandals and a gorgeous lemon-coloured scarf around her neck. She looked stunning.

I noticed that Staff A was carrying her bag for her. Great. So, my ancient mother had to carry hers herself, but old skinny legs was given a helping hand. Immediately, for no reason at all, I got a sudden feeling that something was going on between Staff A and the glamorous brunette. Something about the way he was talking to her...leaning in so closely and smiling. It was the first time I'd seen him smile since we arrived.

And what was someone so skinny doing on a weight loss retreat in the first place? Why would she need to be here? It didn't add up.

He helped her into the minibus with such tenderness, it was like a scene from Love Story. "Everything OK?" he asked. "Just say if you need anything." Then he stroked her cheek gently and closed the doors.

"Let's go," he said to Staff B.

"I'm Yvonne," said the attractive lady and we all murmured greetings back to her as she made herself comfortable, taking up about 1 inch of space.

"Have you known Staff A long," I said.

"No, I've never met him before," she said.

"Oh, you two seemed so close. I assumed you were old friends."

"Nope, we've never met," Staff A added quickly, shouting over from his position in the front seat. "Now make sure you all do up your seatbelts."

"She clicked hers around her and sort smiled at me, putting out a delicate hand for me to shake. I was struggling to get the seat belt done up, it simply wouldn't go around me so I abandoned it and put my hand out to shake hers. In horror, I realised that my hand was about four times the size of hers. Her tiny, delicate little pink nails looked like those of a child next to my hands which look like shovels.

God, life was so depressing. I think my hands were bigger than hers when I was born. Hands and feet are things that are not supposed to be big if you're a woman.

At times like these, I long to be delicate, small and adorable. Or, if the truth be known, I'd settle for being more attractive than my mother. That shouldn't be too much for a woman to ask for, should it?

The journey to the villas we were staying in for the retreat took around an hour and a half in boiling sunshine. There was air-conditioning in the vehicle, but it was certainly nothing like strong enough to prevent us all feeling weak with the heat.

"Is there any chance you could turn the air-conditioning up a bit?" I asked.

"You're going to have to get used to this heat lady, you're going to be exercising in this all day every day for the rest of the week," said Staff A.

God how I wanted to punch him.

"She's right though, it is terribly hot, is there anything you can do?" said Yvonne.

"Let me have a look," he said. He fiddled with the dials at the front, and when he couldn't make the air-conditioning any colder, he handed her his notebook and advised her to fan herself. I looked from him to her and back again, and felt like the most unimportant, ugly person on Earth.

WE ARRIVED at the health camp (I shall insist on calling it that, even though it's a 'military fitness camp') after baking in the minivan and stepped out onto a street of pretty chalk-coloured houses. In the middle of the row of attractive homes in yellow, soft blue and pink, were four red brick houses. "There are Villa 1, Villa 2, Villa 3 and Villa 4," said Staff B. "You are all in Villa 3. Please note that all food is served in Villa 1 and all classes and walks start from Villa 1. That is the main base of the activities. You are all free to go into any of the villas, but your bedrooms are in Villa 1. The keys to each of the villas are kept under the large stones outside the front doors. Once you've let yourself in, please replace the key so that the next person can also let themselves in. If you accidentally take the key with you, you'll cause chaos. Also, the bedrooms don't lock, so you won't need a lock for them. You'll find it's quite safe. Understand?"

We all nodded to indicate our understanding, but it wasn't enough for grumpy Staff A.

"What was that?" he asked, turning around.

We all murmured that yes, that was fine.

"When you're asked a question, you respond with 'yes staff'. OK?"

"Yes staff," we all said.

"And you understand that you mustn't move the key from under the rock?"

"Yes staff," we all said.

"OK then, let's go."

It was a beautiful place, very quiet and with these lovely bright orange and red flowers popping out all over the place - in baskets outside the villa and even from between the cracks in the wall.

"Come to Villa 1 at 5pm," said Staff B. "We'll run through the programme for the rest of the week and then go for a quick walk before dinner. OK?"

"Yes, staff," we all replied, as I bounced my case and mum's bag down the old stone steps towards the front door of the villa. I noticed that Yvonne had gone off with Staff A and Staff B. Definitely something fishy going on there.

WALKING AND FAINTING

After the drama of the soldiers frog marching us to the minibus and the shock of discovering that my mother is way more fanciable than I am, it was a relief to open the door to the villa and discover that it was gorgeous inside...really lovely. There was a central seating area with three large sofas around a television, a large balcony with a table and chairs on it, and a good-sized kitchen complete with washing machine.

The room that mum and I were sharing was downstairs, so I lugged the two bags down the 12 steps and pushed open the door to the room.

When I looked inside, I gasped with relief. I was half expecting bunk beds and camouflage-patterned duvet covers with khaki towels, and no running water, but it was like a lovely hotel room. The best thing was the floor to ceiling glass doors that swept open onto a patio, with a swimming pool beyond.

"Oh my," said mum. "This looks lovely."

We dumped our bags on the beds and opened the patio doors before walking out to the pool where Simon and Graham were standing, staring into the water.

Karen walked over to join us. She had very short dark hair that was cut like a man's hair, and quite big features. She wasn't unattractive, just not 'pretty' much to my relief.

"Thank God!" she said as she arrived next to us. "I was worried that the rooms were going to be set up like a military dorm after seeing those two nutters who picked us up from the airport."

"Me too," I squealed, rather louder than I meant to. I was just so excited that the room was a proper hotel room and not a terrible army base. I was also pleased that she seemed as disconcerted by the army stuff as I was. I didn't want to be the only person on the camp who didn't know it was run by the army.

"I don't think I was made for soldiering," she said. "I'm just not good at being shouted at."

"Gosh, me neither," I said. "I hate it when people should at me. And look at the size of this arse - I was not built for running around all over the place."

Karen smiled and laughed, and in that moment an unlikely bond was created between Karen and me, a bond built on mutual dislike of khaki and mud and a solidarity to avoid all military-related activity at all costs.

She high fived me and I smiled warmly. I'd made a friend. Not the sort of friend who'd be with me for a lifetime, but someone who'd help keep me sane over the coming days.

The only downside of chatting away to Karen was that I had left mum at the mercy of Simon. I looked round as she giggled girlishly. Simon looked away as I gave him the death stare that I normally save for customers in the DIY centre who move all the plants to the wrong places.

Simon scurried off and mum came to join me as we sat on the recliners, next to the pool and soaked up the remainder of the afternoon's sunshine. It was heaven...blue skies, a glistening pool and a couple of hours in which to relax.

We'd been told to meet in villa number one at 5pm and it was 3pm now. From there we would all go for a walk before dinner. It all seemed reassuringly civilised. I had a nice room, I'd made a nice friend and now I was going on a walk before dinner. Perhaps this whole thing would be OK after all?

I drifted off to sleep until mum woke me up at quarter to five. As soon as I opened my eyes I was absolutely starving. The sun was still beating down on me. I needed a very large gin and tonic and a very large burger and fries.

"Are we eating before going on the walk?" I asked.

"I don't think so," she replied. She'd changed into the gym gear that we bought in Sports Direct and looked like she was about to race in the Olympic 100m event.

I staggered out of the sunshine and into the cool haven of my room. I hadn't unpacked and really couldn't be bothered to.

"Do you think I'll be OK in these sandals?" I asked mum. "I can't be bothered to unpack my whole case to get my trainers out."

"Well, obviously trainers would be better," she responded, "but it's only a light evening walk so I'm sure you'll be fine in those on the first night."

So we headed upstairs in the villa, then strode up the stone steps onto the main road and headed down to villa one.

The main villa was very similar in layout to ours, but a little bit bigger, and a bit more bedraggled, if the truth be known. Perhaps it was the fact that so many people sat on the sofas in that villa because it was where everyone congregated meaning everything looked more worn and tired. In our villa we had lovely, plump cream sofas, whereas here they were bedraggled orange ones, with a range of mismatching scatter cushions. I much preferred our villa. Mum and I hovered on the edge of the main room, peering in, unsure whether we should just enter.

"Come in, come in," said a very thin, very fit looking woman, emerging from a side room: you must be from the Two Fat Ladies blog? I'm Abigail."

"Yes, I'm from Two Fat Ladies. I'm Mary," I said. "This is my mum."

"Hello there, nice to meet you," she said. "I really hope you enjoy yourself over the next few days. I'm sure you'll get a lot out of it."

Then she glanced at mum: "You're not fat at all. You look great," she said.

"Thank you, how kind," said mum, blushing.

I know Abi's right, mum does look great, but it still felt like a dagger through me that I was absolutely as fat as she expected but mum wasn't. I know I look fat, but I still find it very hard when I realise that other people see me as fat, or when I'm made to feel fat.

After the pleasantries (or 'unpleasantries' in my case), we all went for what they laughing called an evening stroll. Trades Descriptions Act anyone? My idea of an evening stroll is a gentle, enjoyable walk at a sensible pace.

Their idea of an evening stroll is trying to break some sort of imaginary world record even if it means killing everyone in the group. I tried to keep up, I really did, but the combined forces of strappy sandals, gross unfitness and a body which is twice as large as it should be, prevented me from finishing anywhere near the others. I was about 20 minutes behind them. It was ridiculous, absolutely ridiculous.

"Come on," mum said, in the end, "I could have done the walk five times while you've done it once."

"OK, OK," I said. "Just relax. It's day one, no point in wearing yourself out when we've only just started. I'm saving myself for later in the week."

The simple truth, of course, was that I was going as fast as I possibly could, and it was the fastest they were likely to see me all week, if - indeed - I could tolerate staying all week.

By the time I got back to the villa I felt more exhausted than I ever have in my life before. I was also completely starving and really thirsty.

"Water?" said Staff B, handing me a beaker. I just nodded at him. I'd completely lost the power of speech.

I was aware that I would be absolutely scarlet and soaking wet with sweat - I always was after exercise, but this time I felt much worse than I usually do. I could feel my head spinning, and kept staggering as I stood there. My knees buckled a bit but I managed to gain my composure. I'd be fine in a minute. I sipped on the water, and waited to feel whole again.

"Are you sure you're OK?" asked mum. "You really don't look very well."

"Of course I am," I said, once my voice had come back and I'd stopped shaking.

"You're absolutely bright red you know."

"Yes, I do that when I'm tired," I said. "I'm feeling much better now."

As I spoke, I felt everything spin. I felt all unsteady. I heard mum's shout but it all sounded so far away, I remembered grabbing hold of something that fell to the ground, making a massive sound, and I remember trying to apologise as I hit the deck, then I don't really remember anything else.

AN INCIDENT WITH DONALD

"She's moving.... she's opening her eyes..."
I could hear mum's voice floating above me,
"Can you hear me love?" she was saying. "Clap if you can hear me."

I moved my hands in a clapping motion and made the tiniest sound - the most pathetic sound in the history of clapping. There was a great cheer and everyone in the room started clapping too. I looked up to see them all looking down at me, applauding my attempt at a clap, their faces full of pride at my achievement. I felt like a toddler who'd just used the potty for the first time.

"Are you feeling alright," said a familiar voice.

"Um, yes, I think," I said vaguely. "Is that you, mum?"

"Yes, darling, it's me," she said.

"Where am I?" I couldn't work out where on earth I was. The people looking down at me looked familiar, but they weren't my friends. Who were they? Why were they here, in my bedroom?

"You're at the weight loss camp, remember?" said mum. "We went for a long walk earlier and you couldn't keep up, then you came back and just fell to the ground."

"Oh God, yes. The weight loss camp. Oh God. I wish I hadn't asked."

"We're all about to have supper. Perhaps it'll help you if we get some food inside you...what do you think?" said a male voice, before Staff B's face loomed into view. He smiled at me, and given his position above me, looking down at me, all I could think of was sex. He looked particularly gorgeous from that angle. I knew I needed to move before I pulled him down on top of me and started dry humping him.

"Food sounds like a good idea," I said, sitting up and looking at the faces around me. They all looked so concerned.

"Come and sit down," said Karen. "See if you feel better after dinner."

I was helped to my feet by the two 'staffs' and led to the end of the wooden table. The others came over to join me.

"Sit here," Staff B said, pulling out a wooden chair with his gloved hand (still wearing gloves? Very odd) and seating me.

"I'll bring out the food now. Does everyone else want to sit down as well," said Abigail, wiggling her way into the kitchen, giving us all a sight of her peachy derriere clad in expensive lycra.

I continued to sip the beaker of water, and smiled as a bowl was laid before me. I peered inside it and looked at mum. She was nodding at me with a look of victory on her face. The bowl contained orange liquid. She was right. We'd been here just a few hours and already they were serving us bloody carrots.

DINNER DIDN'T TAKE TOO LONG, as you can probably imagine. Boiled, mashed carrots don't demand a lot of chewing. I finished and waited patiently for something else...anything else - even a celery stick or an apple would have been nice - you know - something to chew on, get my teeth into. But that was it. Just a bowl full of carroty baby food.

"That was actually quite filling, wasn't it?" said Yvonne, helping me to my feet and asking whether I was OK.

She led me over to the orange sofas and sat me down gently. Everyone else had sat down too. There were about 20 of us on the course, five in each villa. There were people of all shapes and sizes, but none as shapely as me. They all seemed very kind and genuinely concerned about me, which was nice, even Simon the mother-stalker handed me a cushion and asked whether I needed anything.

I sat back into the sofa and felt quite relaxed. It had been a dramatic start to the trip, but the people were all nice, the accommodation was lovely and if I ate like that, I'd lose about 40 stone by the end of the week, so it wasn't all bad.

"Shall we play a game," said a guy with ginger hair and a rather unflattering ginger goatee beard. I didn't know the guy at all. I knew his name was Mark because he'd introduced himself to me on the walk earlier, but he wasn't in our villa so I knew nothing about him. I liked him though. He had been kind enough to offer to stay back and keep me company on the walk earlier while the others had stormed ahead like they were heading into battle.

"Yes, a game sounds good," I replied, more because I thought he was a nice guy so wanted to support him than because I have any interest at all in playing games.

"Yes," said another guy I didn't know. "If there's no eating or drinking allowed this evening, a game would be a good distraction."

"OK," said Mark. "I'm going to pose a question then we have to go around the room and all answer it. It'll help us to get to know one another as well. Make sure you say your name before you answer."

I was slightly concerned about this - not for my sake - I'm quite outgoing and happy to answer any questions, but mum's so reserved - I knew she wouldn't want to answer any personal questions.

"What's the weirdest memory you have of school?" asked Mark.

Fast as lightning mum's hand shot up.

"I remember a teacher at school being sacked once," she said, laughing as she spoke. "It was so strange...there was an eagle's nest outside and all the children had to go and look at it on Fridays. For some reason it always fell to this particular teacher to take us and she got completely fed up, so one afternoon, when she thought everyone had left the building, she picked up some rocks and hurled them at the nest. It was alarming. I think they were endangered at the time. The birds squawked, the caretaker came and Mrs Thatchmaker was escorted from the building. No one saw her again, nor the eagles. I don't know whether she killed them or terrified them so much that the mummy eagle decided to move them somewhere safer."

I was flabbergasted. Where had mum suddenly got all this confidence from?

"That's so funny. You're a gifted storyteller," said Simon, smiling at mum until he saw me watching him closely and turned away. I swear, if I haven't strangled him by the end of this holiday it will be a bloody miracle.

"How about you, Simon? Do you have a story from your school days?" I asked, hoping to catch him out without a tale to tell.

"Well, I have a rather vivid and disconcerting memory that I could share with you," he said.

"Do go on," said Yvonne.

"In junior school our English teacher would put on a new coat of lipstick in in the brightest red colour, and kiss the boys whenever they misbehaved in class," he said. "Once she'd kissed one of us, we weren't allowed to wipe it off. It happened to me and it was mortifying...I never crossed her again."

"That's rather a good idea," said mum. "Disciplining the boys without resorting to violence. I like that. I might adopt that if anyone crosses me. I'll kiss them on the cheek and that will stop them."

"Now I really want to cross you," said Simon, smiling lasciviously at mum, causing everyone in the room to look slightly awkward.

"Right, on that note, I'm going to head off to bed. Are you coming, mum?"

"Oh. Actually, I thought I might stay here for a little while and play this game," she said. "Why don't you stay and join in?"

"I just need to get some sleep," I said, though - in truth - I had a little snack secreted in my bag, and I needed to eat it before I died of hunger.

"I'll come and walk you back," said mum.

"No, no - you stay. I'll be fine. It takes about 10 seconds to get back. I'll see you later."

"See you in the morning," said Karen, offering a friendly wave.

"I'll walk out with you - I'm heading out," said Yvonne, leaning over to help me to my feet.

"Where are you going?" I asked, hoping upon hope that she was heading out to the pub. If she was going to a pub, I was definitely going with her. I really needed a drink; I wanted to do an 'Aunty Susan', and drink and eat my way through the evening.

"I've found a lovely hotel on the seafront with a great gym with a sauna and spa. I'm going to do a quick work out and sit in the sauna before bed."

"Really?" I said. It baffled me that anyone would want to do extra exercise. "Don't overdo it though - we've got loads on tomorrow without you trying to squeeze in any extra voluntary stuff tonight."

"I won't overdo it" she said. "See you later."

She walked away in shorts so tight they must have been stitched on by her gynaecologist.

I loitered near the door for a minute, listening to mum and the others still telling their stories. "Come on, a few more silly tales," mum was saying. "I'm enjoying this. Actually, I remember something my husband told me. It's a very funny story; he was in his science class and the teacher was introducing them to the subject of electricity. The teacher told the whole class to hold hands, with the children on the end holding a generator. He was going to give them a little tingle of electricity and demonstrate how humans conducted it as it went all along the line of children. But the teacher had it turned up way too high and he electrocuted half of them. Your father was in hospital for a week and had terrible burns on his hands."

"Oh, my goodness," said Staff B, joining the group. "Did that happen to you?"

"No, my husband," said mum.

He looked over at me. "How are you feeling now?"

"OK," I said. "I was just leaving. I feel really tired."

"You should get an early night. If you're not feeling right tomorrow, I'll call a doctor and we'll get him to take a look at you."

"OK," I said. "I'm sure I'll be fine, I just over did it."

"All the more reason to get an early night then," said Staff B. "Do you want me to walk with you?"

"No, I'll be fine," I said. "Karen, would you mind making sure mum gets back safely?"

"Of course," she said. "No problem at all."

"Thank you. Good night everyone," I said, heading through the door as they resumed their game and told silly stories about their time at school. It was only a few steps back to the villa - I walked up the stone steps, through the gate, along to the next villa, down the steps and took the key from under the stone, I let myself in and walked down to the bedroom. It had seemed odd that the rooms didn't lock when I first arrived, but now it was a Godsend - I just pushed the door open, wandered inside and slumped onto the bed. I couldn't be bothered to unpack my suitcase and find my nightie, so I just stripped off, dumped my phone on the bedside cabinet and climbed between the sheets. I fell fast asleep as soon as my head touched the pillow.

AND, to be fair, that's exactly where I would have stayed had it not been for the feel of someone getting into the bed next to me and jumping back out again.

"Who the hell are you?" said a male voice.

I hastily pushed the light on and there stood a man in his 60s in his Y-fronts. I recognised him from earlier but didn't know his name. I certainly hadn't invited him to join me.

"Get out of my room," I screamed, wrapping the duvet around me as I sat up. "Get out."

"This is my room," said the man.

"This is not your room. It's my room. I share it with my mum."

"Look around," he said. "I've got all my stuff here…see…. You're very welcome to stay, but it's not your room."

He was right. His things were laid out on the dressing table, his trainers were neatly by the long mirror. There was no sign of my unpacked suitcase anywhere. Nor any sign of mum.

"Oh shit," I said, wrapping his sheet around me and gathering my clothes together. "I don't know how this happened."

"This is villa two," he said. He was staring at my body, not looking at my face while I spoke to him.

"Oh God, I'm villa three," I said. "I'll be off now."

"No, stay," he said. "Why don't you stay here. I can look after you. I'm Donald, by the way."

"Err, no thanks. I'm going," I said, and I ran from the room, ran up the stairs and into the right room in the right villa. Thankfully mum wasn't back yet, so I climbed into the right bed and fell asleep.

Jesus Christ, Mary, great start to the trip.

SWING YOUR ARMS, MARY

The alarm clock burst into life at 5.30am and mum leapt out of bed like a wild salmon. "Come on, up you get," she said. "Remember we've got our walk this morning before breakfast."

"A walk? You're joking, right? Were you not there for that walk last night? It was a travesty. We must've done about 20 miles. It almost killed me. Perhaps I shouldn't come this morning?"

"Gosh you do exaggerate, you'll be fine, just remember to wear your trainers and drink lots of water," said mum pulling back the floor-to-ceiling curtains and letting a most unwelcome flash of early morning light into the room. The pool in the courtyard was glittering in the morning sunshine, just outside the patio doors.

"Oh my God - I've just remembered something," I said, staring at the pool. "Last night…something really weird happened."

"What?" asked mum. "When I got in, you were fast asleep."

"Yes - before that. Oh God."

Mum was looking at me intently but I couldn't find the words to explain to her.

"What happened?" she asked, all wide-eyed, dressed in nothing but her sports bra and an offensively large pair of pants.

"I fainted," I said, "I just remembered that I fainted."

She didn't need to know that I'd jumped into the bed of a 60-year-old called Donald.

"Yes, you did," she said kindly. "Are you feeling OK now?"

"Much better," I said.

I clambered out of bed and started to look around for my phone. I couldn't see it anywhere. I got that horrible lurching feeling in the pit of my stomach that appeared whenever I couldn't find my phone.

"Shit."

I tipped out the contents of my handbag and wracked my brain.

"What on earth's the matter?" asked mum. "What have you lost?"

"My phone. I don't know what I've done with it."

"You probably left it in villa one last night. Let's check when we get there. Or maybe it fell out of your pocket when you fainted?"

"Yes, probably," I said. "Maybe I should look for my phone instead of the walk? I could catch up with you all later?"

"No, you're coming on the walk," said mum. "We've come all this way to get fit and healthy…this is a great chance for you to lose some weight and start to feel good. It's silly to start missing out on things on day one."

"OK, OK," I said. "I'll come on the walk, but you have to be aware that if it's anything like last night's walk, it will kill me and there's every chance that you'll be arrested for murder for making me go on it."

"The walk last night was about five miles, that's all, and it was very nice. All the people we met were lovely, and the scenery was spectacular. Come on, up you get. We're walking along the beach this morning, then hopefully we'll have time to come back and jump in that pool afterwards. Doesn't it look spectacular? Just spectacular."

"I knew it was a mistake bringing you," I said, as I staggered like a drunk into the bathroom. Why couldn't my mum be miserable in the mornings like everyone else on earth? As I clambered into the shower, I could hear her singing to herself as she got changed. God, the backs of my legs were aching. The truth was that I was so bloody unfit that every bit of exercise we did was going to render me feeling exhausted and in pain. Mum, on the other hand, was a regular walker, played a bit of tennis, and did a lot of gardening. In short, she was about 30 years older than me but twice as fit as me. And if that wasn't an embarrassing prospect, I thought to myself as I washed my hair and clambered out of the shower, I didn't know what was.

I followed mum out of the room, my hair was still wet and my unforgiving gym kit made me feel the size of a house. We walked to villa one where we were all meeting. I shuffled along in a sulk, staring at the ground while mum strode ahead, and shouted 'morning' to everyone she encountered. I decided I was not saying good morning to anyone.

"Mary, Mary," came a shout from a man running towards us. I gasped when I saw him. It was Donald - the guy from last night...the guy who had come into his room and seen me in fast-asleep in his bed. Oh God. In his hand he held my phone.

"You left this is my room," he said. I looked at him aghast, alarm spreading across my face like an uncontrollable rash. He mistook my alarm for confusion. "When you were in my bed last night. Remember? Well, you left this behind."

I looked at mum who was open-mouthed.

"It's not how it looks," I mouthed. "I went into his bed by mistake."

Mum's mouth was still wide open.

"IT WAS A MISTAKE."

"I'll say it was," she said. "Having an affair with an older man on holiday when you have such a lovely boyfriend at home...a huge mistake."

"Mum, I didn't have an affair. I went to the wrong villa, that's all. They all look the same, the doors aren't locked. It was an easy mistake to make."

Mum looked at me and shook her head.

"Do you really think I would cheat on Ted?" I said. "Ted is the nicest man in the world, I'd never do anything to upset him, you must know that."

"Of course I do. I'm just teasing you."

We both looked up and saw Staff B ahead, warning up by bending over in perilously tight shorts. "One word of advice though, Mary. If you do decide to get into a man's bed accidentally, get into the bed of a man like Staff B, not dopey Donald, won't you."

"Will do," I said as Staff B stood up. He had on the shortest shorts, but still wore a long-sleeved t-shirt and those white gloves he seemed obsessed with. He was stubbly and muscular and oozed masculinity. Mum was right. That would definitely have been a better bed to have found myself in.

"Ready for our little morning walk," he said, giving me a gentle hug. "You don't have to look so sad. It's only a quick stroll along the beach."

"I'm not sad," I said. "I just don't believe you. It won't be a quick walk at all: I'm wise to your madness now. I'm well aware that when you say a quick walk along the beach you mean that we're going to do an Ironman triathlon in world record beating time."

"Not quite," he said with a warm laugh. "It's just a morning stroll to knock away the cobwebs."

He grinned as he walked away but I knew he was lying. 'Stroll'? Really? I didn't think it would be at all stroll-ish.

I went and sat on the small stone wall outside the villa while everyone else warmed up. I knew I should join in, but I felt so self-conscious, so I sat and focused on the lovely purple flowers growing out of the rocks next to us, gently cupping one of them in my hand and making a mental note to find out what they were, they were so beautiful - like tiny pansies with lovely, open faces. I looked up to see Donald watching me and I felt myself blush as I looked away. How could I have been so bloody stupid?

Everyone else was ready to go, some of them jogging on the spot and waving their arms around, some starting to stretch their calves out like they were bloody Paula Radcliffe or something. Then it was time to leave...

We all walked down the street, quite fast. Much faster than I would've chosen to do had I been walking by myself, I had to do little skippy steps to keep up with them. We then went down along the line of steps which led to the beach. "Come on, let's get a bit of speed up shall we," said Staff B, jogging down them, then sprinting out

43

across the sand. Oh Christ. I just wasn't fit enough to do any of this, as I ran down the steps, I could feel my boobs bouncing up and down and my stomach moving like it had a mind of its own. Instinctively I pulled my t-shirt down and held it flat against my body as if to disguise the horrible flesh beneath it. I hated being fat. Being fat was horrible.

"What's up with you?" said Staff B. "You look like you're really fed up. Look at your mum, she's out there jogging along the beach."

"You said it would be a walk," I bit back.

I looked up to see mum running along with the others. They were lifting their knees up as high as they could and had their arms out in front of them so that their knees were tapping against their hands. They were already miles in front.

"I can't do any of this because I'm too fat," I said, disconsolately. "It hurts when I run and skip and jump."

"Well, just walk then. The important thing is to keep moving."

"I'm not going to lose all this weight by walking, am I?" I said.

"Yes, of course you will. If you vow to move whenever you can, however you want, you'll lose the weight. It's not rocket science."

"But it will take years of effort and I haven't got the motivation for it."

"You don't need motivation. Stop thinking of exercising as some sort of horrible punishment. Look, this is how I see it. First thing - speed up a little bit and walk next to me. That's not too bad, is it? Walking at this speed where you can feel yourself getting out of breath will use a lot more calories."

"OK, I can do that," I said.

"Now, swing your arms as you walk," he said. I swung them by my side. "See how fast you can swing them," he said. I swung them backwards and forwards as quickly as I could and noticed that my pace was speeding up.

"A little tip for you there, Mary," he said. "You will find that your legs will go as fast as your arms are swinging, so if you want to make yourself go faster just swing your arms faster and your legs will keep up. If you walk along like you have been doing with your arms hardly swinging at all, you will find that you automatically walk more slowly."

"Good tip," I said.

"And you know what you've just been saying to me about losing weight?"

"Yes," I said, hoping he was going to give me some magical formula for losing weight that would enable me to shift 10 stone this week.

"I think you need to stop thinking about it as being all about weight loss. Yes, you want to lose weight, but you want weight loss to be the by-product of what you do to get yourself feeling fit healthy and wonderful.

"I think the what you need to focus on is looking after yourself a bit more. So, don't put anything in your mouth that isn't going to do you good. Drink lots of water because it will stop you having headaches and make you feel full of energy, and just use your legs and your body as much as you can because being fit is the key to feeling great.

"All you are doing from now onwards is looking after yourself and trying to feel as great and wonderful as possible.

"Stop trying to tick off the number of pounds you've lost, and stop mentally totting up how many months it's going to be before you meet some arbitrary desired weight. Just take each day as it comes and, on that day, do everything you can to make yourself feel and look better. How about that as a plan?"

The arm swinging seemed to be working well, and I had almost caught up with the rest of the group who were busy doing star jumps on the side of the beach near the cliff.

"Okay, I can do that," I said. "Thank you."

He leaned in and gave me a big hug and said: "You know, Mary Brown, it's all going to be okay. You're young, attractive, and prepared to do something to make yourself fitter and healthier. You've got a lovely life ahead of you - you've just got to believe that."

"I believe," I said in a loud, mock American accent, being sarcastic with him as he smiled and walked away, but the truth was that I did feel quite good, better than I had for ages, and I did feel as if I believed

I could do something about the way I looked. I smiled at his retreating back and thought. "This could be the best week of my life."

Then I saw Donald approaching, clutching a small purple flower like the ones I'd been admiring earlier. "Hello bed mate," he said, with an unattractive wink. "Thought you might like this…"

WEIGHTS AND MEASURES

"Right, let's get going on with the weighing and measuring," said Staff A, clapping his hands and rubbing them together. "We want to make sure that you know exactly where you are beginning of the course so you can see how much you progress in just a few days."

This struck me as odd. Hadn't Staff B just spent 10 minutes having an emotional chat with me on the beach in which he said that I shouldn't focus on weight?"

I couldn't resist mentioning this...in the hope that they would abandon their plans to weigh us.

"Yes, Mary, that's true," he said, a hint of exasperation sneaking into the corners of his voice. "But this is to help you see what impact we can have when we work really hard. It's a motivational tool more than anything else. Does that make sense?"

"Yes," I said. Though it didn't really. I didn't understand why a course which decried the process of weighing and measuring, weighed and measured us all at the beginning and the end of the course.

I think he could sense that I was still very confused. "OK, I can see that it seems odd," he said. "I wouldn't advise worrying too much about your weight, look at how you look and how you feel and what makes you happy rather than what random numbers on a scale tell you.

"We are all different builds, all different makeups, the idea that everybody who is 5'6" should weigh the same is simply wrong, but it's a useful guide to see how you've changed over the course."

I nodded at him, realising that I wasn't going to get out of this and they were going to measure me regardless. I suppose the weighing gives them a handy marketing tool: 'lose half a stone in four days' is a lot more exciting a proposition than 'get a bit healthier, but not measurably so because we don't believe in measuring and weighing.'

I was first up. That would teach me to answer back to the instructor. I stepped onto the scales and watched the numbers in front of me rising with astounding speed, getting bigger and bigger until they settled on… 20 stone and 4 pounds.

"That's wrong!" I squealed, jumping off as if the thing had bitten me. I saw the looks of horror on the faces of those waiting in the dining room for their turn to be measured. A bit like that time I screamed in the dentists at such blood-curdling volume that the waiting room had cleared by the time I came out.

"I can't possibly be that heavy. That's the weight a baby elephant should be, or a car or something, not a human being."

"Don't worry about it," said Staff A with a smile. "It's just a number. It just tells you where you are now, and then we can see where you are at the end of the week, and work out what changes have taken place."

"But to be over 20 stone…that's insane," I said. "Your scales are drunk."

"Twenty stone!" squealed mum. "That can't be right can it?"

"No!" I shouted back. "It most certainly isn't."

"You told me you were 15 stone."

"I am," I said. "The scales are wrong."

I looked at Staff A. "The scales are right, aren't they?" I said miserably.

"Yep," he said. "But try not to worry. You're in the right place with the right people I will help you sort all this out. OK?"

"Yes," I said.

I walked back to mum.

"That can't be right," she said.

"No," I said, shaking my head vigorously.

"So, the scales were wrong?" she asked.

"Yes," I said. "They hadn't set them up properly."

"So, how heavy are you?" asked mum.

"Fifteen stone," I replied.

Mum went on next and came skipping back to declare that she was 10 and half stone. "I'm really pleased because I thought my weight was creeping up towards 11 stone."

"Yes, that would have been awful," I said, uncharitably, while I chewed on the fact that mum was about half my weight.

It took a little while for the whole weighing process to happen, so we were treated to a film to keep us entertained while they did it. Not a film in the way you or I might recognise it - no Sex & The City or Bridesmaids or anything, just a film about being healthy and getting fit. And no popcorn, of course. Not even the naff plain stuff that I accidentally buy sometimes by mistake when I'm aiming for the toffee coated stuff.

Staff B stepped up to sort out the video, and after a considerable amount of trouble connecting his laptop to the large screen, including him showing everyone all his emails, he appeared to have asserted some sort of technological control.

"Phew," he said. "That was harder than I thought it would be. OK. Before we start on today's sessions, and while the weighing is going on, we have a quick video to show you. Before I do that, a quick question - who was alarmed by their weight and is disappointed at weighing more than they thought they would?"

Loads of hands shot up, including bone-skinny Yvonne's which really annoyed me. I bet her weight hardly registered on the scale.

"Well, I want you to stop worrying - the reason for us weighing you is just to show you that if you eat right and exercise well, you WILL lose weight. But we'd very much like you to park the whole weight issue.

"As staff explained to Mary earlier, we mustn't put too much emphasis on how much we weigh. What's important is how you feel, and to most of you it'll be how you look. I'm sure you'd much rather look great in a dress than hit a particular weight measurement but not look great. Isn't that right?"

"Yes," we all chorused.

"And how are you all feeling today?"

"Fat!" I shouted, while everyone else shouted "great."

THE VIDEO SHIMMERED into life and a rather sombre-looking guy, dressed in a white coat like a doctor or scientist, appeared on the screen.

"Obesity is such a problem that we spend more on it than on the fire service, the police service and the judiciary all put together," he said.

Sighs of disbelief drifted in from all corners of the room.

"It's alarming isn't it?" he continued. "It shows what a problem it is. And it also shows how hard it is to deal with - do you know why that is? Why don't we all just eat less?

"The reason is in our biology - it's because we are forcing ourselves to live a life that suits our minds, not our bodies. We have bodies that are designed to store food and a brain that is designed to be attracted to food - these are survival instincts that worked when food was scarce. But now we're living in a part of the world where there's plenty of food while these instincts remain.

"So - what you're all wondering is - what do we do about it? These facts might help to give you a clue: we are now 20% less active than we were back in the 1960s. Exercise is a vital part of good health."

There were mumblings of agreement and I mumbled along with them but to be honest, I don't think exercise is the key to anything but abject misery.

"Exercise is one of five things you need to do to lose weight. Numerous investigations have shown this. These are the five things: eat less, exercise more, drink water when you're hungry, remember that your body was designed for times when there was no food around and it had to carefully conserve everything you put into it, and – finally - walk, walk and walk again."

I was starting to get really frustrated with the whole thing. If I could 'eat less' I wouldn't be obese in the first place.

"There are lots of diets being promoted all the time," science man was continuing. "Lots of them marketed as the answer to all your weight loss problems. But there are real issues associated with opting for the latest fad diet, or the diet that appears to be 'proven' to be the best way to lose weight. Let me demonstrate."

Suddenly science man was standing in front of a university.

"So, a study, conducted at this university, found that low-carb dieters fared much better than those who followed a low-fat diet and showed better results on blood tests that indicate cardiovascular health.

"Then a few months later, a University of South Carolina study published in the International Journal of Applied and Basic Nutritional Sciences found the greatest weight loss was found on a high-carbohydrate vegan diet.

So, within two months, the evidence points to the fact that low-carb diets work, and high-carb diets work.

"There have been reports that depression and obesity are strongly linked, that eating breakfast helps you lose weight, and then, a few months later, further research to show that none of that is true.

"The reason I'm saying all this is to show you that having a healthy scepticism about studies is important. Some are good, some are bad. Even the good ones can be overturned with another study a few years on."

The video ended with a montage of good old-fashioned advice about eating a healthy, balanced diet: Don't eat too much, drink lots of water and avoid mood-altering foods like sugar-laden drinks, cakes and coffee that send your hormones into overdrive."

"So, what do you all think of that?" said Staff B.

No one spoke, so I thought I ought to.

"Oh God. It's all so complicated," I said.

"Exactly. The point is that if you try to do fad diet plans or exercise regimes, or try to miss out one food group in an effort to shed the pounds, you are unlikely to achieve a good result long term. If you keep it simple and follow our advice - not only will you look better, but you'll all be much healthier. Does that make sense?"

"Yes," I said. It did make sense. I was sick of following stupid diet fads. I would give this a go."

"Good. So, on that note, let me introduce you to today's activities."

He pulled out a blackboard that was full of classes. I swear to God, there were 10 on there.

"Are you having a laugh?" I asked, more loudly than I intended to.

"You don't have to do all the classes," said Staff A, but you'll get a much better result if you do everything."

"The result will be me in intensive care," I said.

"No one wants that," said the instructor. "Just do whatever you can and try to push yourself as much as possible."

I sensed that my constant talking back at him was starting to wear a bit thin. Still, the blackboard. You should have bloody seen it: First was boxing, then circuits, then cycling, followed by swimming and that was all before lunch. In the afternoon something called heat, followed by body combat, body conditioning, body pump and Pilates, then more boxing. JESUS CHRIST

"Before all that, though - breakfast," he said.

Possibly the only sensible thing anyone has said since I arrived in this God-forsaken place.

STAFF B COMES TO VISIT

The day was exhausting. I mean - terrifyingly tiring, and I only did half of it. I opted for missing out every other class so that I could cope with it all. The day was to end with a final boxing class held on the top of a steep hill, which practically took crampons and advanced mountaineering equipment to climb. I sat on the edge of my bed. Would it really be so bad if I didn't go? I'd missed the first boxing class in the morning, but in my defence, I had been to more classes that day than I'd been to in the previous year, and there were two more days to go. Surely I could miss this one out?

Under the pretence of looking for my water bottle, I told mum to go on ahead and I'd join her.

"OK," she said, smiling and dancing out of the room. Honestly, she's indefatigable.

As soon as she had gone, I flopped onto the bed and experienced a moment of utter joy and exhilaration, lying there, eyes closed, with the sun warming me through the patio windows. Without moving from my position on the bed I eased off my trainers, pushing down the back of the heel with my other foot, and hearing the gentle plop as it hit the floor. I did the same with the other trainer and lay back about as comfortable as any woman has ever been in her life before.

As I felt myself slinking into the bed, and dropping off to sleep, I heard a gentle knock at the door. It must be mum. She must've realised that I wasn't coming and had come back for me. "I'm too tired for boxing," I shouted. "I'm going to have a little sleep before dinner."

It wasn't mum's voice that replied but a deep male voice. "Can I come in? It's Staff B."

I sat up in the bed, ran my hands through my hair and adjusted my clothing to look as alluring as possible. Well, as alluring as a 20 and a half stone woman can look in lycra when she's been exercising all day. I cursed myself for not having come in and had a shower.

"Of course," I said. I arranged myself as seductively as possible, my head resting against my hand, my arm bent, one leg over the other as I lay on my side, in the hope that I would look feminine and elegant.

"Hello there," he said, walking inside and taking a seat in the chair next to my bed. "Everything okay?"

"Yes, fine," I said. "I just feel completely knackered. I couldn't face boxing. I'm also weak with hunger. I just don't cope very well without food."

"Well that's what I wanted to talk to you about," said Staff B. "You didn't come along for the snack just now before boxing. Everyone else was desperate for it. I figured perhaps you weren't feeling very well?"

"Snack?" I said. "I didn't know there was a snack?"

"Yes." That's when he presented me with a tiny piece of flapjack. Honestly it was minuscule... about the size of my thumbnail, but nothing has ever given me greater pleasure.

"Is this for me?" I asked, as if he just given me a jumbo jet or something.

"All yours," he said. I picked it up off the plate as if it was the most precious thing ever, and put it onto the end of my tongue, determined to make it last as long as possible

"I can't believe I missed a snack," I said to Staff B. "I've never missed a snack in my life before."

He smiled warmly.

"Why aren't you with the boxers?" I asked.

"We're mixing things up - Staff A and Abi are taking this one so I can get a couple of hours off. I've got a bit of paperwork to do, and I'm working the session tomorrow as well as being in charge of the great big martial arts, combat and boxing three-hour marathon session on Thursday morning."

"WHAT?"

"Yep - three hours of boxing, kicking and wrestling. Pure joy."

"Good God this is hardcore," I said. "Why so much boxing and fighting?"

"It's a military fitness camp. What did you think we'd be doing? Needlework?"

"Ha, ha," I said. "Can I ask you something?"

"Fire away," he said.

"Why are you called Staff B? It seems really weird that we can't just call you by your name."

"My name is Martin," he said. "But here they like the instructors to be called staff."

"Why? It's absurd, to insist on everything being so military when we're just a bunch of flabby people wanting to lose a few pounds."

"Yes," he said, with a smile. "But there is a sensible reason. You see – in the army when you're a PT instructor you don't have a rank, you're all called staff, so no one knows what rank you are. The reason for that is that physical fitness is very important, and you couldn't have a situation where the physical trainer is instructing someone of a higher rank, and the person of the higher rank didn't want to do it so pulled rank.

"They decided the best thing was that when it came to physical training everyone involved was just called staff and were all equal."

"Oh, I see, "I said. "That makes sense. I can see why they would do that. Why on earth don't they explain that to us, it would make us all feel much better about the names we have to call you."

"I don't know really," said Staff B. "Maybe I'll mention it to Abi?"

"Did you like it in the army?" I asked.

"I loved it," he said, taking off his boots, putting his feet up on the bed and removing his watch as he made himself comfortable. Interestingly, the gloves stayed on.

"My dad was a soldier and my grandad before him. All of the men in my family end up in the army, it's in the blood. It's all I ever wanted to do, and when I got in the army, I felt like I'd come home. Then there was the tour to Afghanistan where it all went horribly wrong."

"What happened?"

"In short, I had my arm blown off," he said bluntly. "It's why I always wear long-sleeved shirts. Look..." He lifted his shirt sleeve and I could see the prosthetic arm beneath it. I'd never noticed before. He always wore gloves and always wore long sleeves, and no one was anyone the wiser.

"Gosh. Did someone shoot at you? What happened?"

"No, it was a landmine. It was in an area where we knew there were landmines, but I was much further out than we thought they went. Four of us were standing there. One guy died."

"Oh God. I'm so sorry," I said. "How awful"

"Yep," he said, nodding. "All pretty awful. When I left, I had no idea what I'd do with myself. Like I explained - being a soldier was in my blood...I couldn't think how I'd survive without it. Doing military-style training for civilians saved me. I couldn't have gone into an office job or anything, it would have driven me nuts. Or worked in a shop. Can you imagine that? Working in a shop all day..."

"I work in a shop," I said timidly.

"Oh. Sorry," he replied. "I just think it would have driven me insane."

"Don't worry. It drives me insane sometimes," I said. "What about Staff A? Was it the same sort of thing with him? Injured abroad."

Staff B moved to stand up. "No, it was very different with him. I better head off. I'll see you at dinner." With that he was gone, he had deliberately refused to talk about why Staff A had left the army. I knew, instinctively, that there was something odd about this. Staff B's reaction had triggered a little spark of interest in me. Right. That would be my mission. To find out why the guy had left the army and why he had such a close relationship with skinny Yvonne.

It wasn't long before mum came back from boxing looking so bedraggled and exhausted that I was doubly pleased I hadn't gone on the trip up the hill. "What happened to you?" she said, falling onto her bed like a rag doll. "You missed the snack and everything."

"Yes, sorry," I said.

"What's this?" Mum held up Staff B's watch, that he'd left on the edge of her bed.

"Oh yes - that's Staff B's," I said, not quite realising how dodgy that sounded.

She handed me the watch, her eyebrows raised so high they had disappeared into her hairline. "Staff B's," she said. "You know I wasn't serious when I said you should try to bed him next time. You know I was only joking, don't you?"

"Ha ha ha," I said. "You're so funny, mum. Nothing happened. He just came to see me."

"And undressed?"

"No, he didn't undress. He just took his watch off."

"Yep - very likely story," said mum. "Very likely story indeed."

"He dropped my snack off, if you must know. And he wanted to see how I was. I guess he thought it was so unlikely that I would miss the chance of food that he thought there must be something wrong with me."

"So, let's just summarise things so far - on the first night here you end up in Donald's bedroom, and on the second night here Staff B ends up in your bedroom. You're having a good trip so far, aren't you?"

Mum laughed as she said it, and I just shook my head and lay back down on the pillow. There was no point to defending myself when she was in such a silly mood.

"I think all the exercise is making you high," I said. "You're behaving like a drunk teenager. And actually, he told me about his time in the army and how he had to leave because his arm was blown off."

"Blown off?"

"Yep. I've got your attention now, haven't I? His arm was blown off by a landmine so he left. He has an artificial arm."

"Gosh, I've never noticed that before."

"No, but you remember how he always wears long sleeves and gloves? That's why."

"I want to hear more about this," said mum. "I'll have a shower after dinner instead of now. What else did he say?"

"Not much, to be honest. He said that when he left, he didn't know what he'd do with himself...all his family are soldiers and it's all he ever wanted to do. I think this place saved him."

"Gosh, that's incredible. Fancy losing your arm."

Mum had wandered towards the patio windows and was looking at the pool as she spoke.

"Makes you realise how grateful you should be, doesn't it?" she said.

WE WALKED up to dinner together, both of us fantasising about the food that might be on offer. Mum thought it might be a gorgeous Italian meal, a lovely pasta dish with fresh lobster and freshly caught prawns. I said it would probably be a big steak and chips, or maybe a massive American burger with chips covered in chilli con carne.

"Shall we have a big bowl of nachos to start?" Mum said.

"Oh yes," I agreed. "And some of those salt and pepper calamari that are delicious. Maybe we should have a whole big selection of starters, before we get onto our main course."

"Good idea," said mum.

We got into the dining room, salivating with excitement at the thought of the food we had been discussing, then sat down and winced a little as they brought out a bowl of broccoli soup.

"At least it's not carrot," said Mum.

"Oh yes it is," said Abi, appearing beside us. "It's broccoli and carrot."

"Oh good," I said. "Exactly what we were both hoping for."

As soon as dinner was over, I wanted to go back to the room... I had visions of falling into an early sleep. Some of the guys talked about going for a walk, but that just felt like massive self-abuse. Why would you do more exercise? It baffled me.

"What are you up to tonight?" I asked Yvonne, who was sitting opposite me.

"I'm going to head off to the sauna again," she said, standing up and moving to leave the table.

"Actually, do you mind if I come with you?" said Simon, standing up as well.

I was intrigued as to how this would all pan out. I mean, if Yvonne was genuinely going to the gym and sauna and not just using it as an excuse to escape and see Staff A, she'd have no problem with Simon going along with her. I glanced at mum and we both awaited Yvonne's reply with some eagerness.

"Not this time Simon," said Yvonne. She smiled at him and left the room at top speed. Minutes later, I was chatting to mum, sitting just across from Staff A, when he jumped up.

"Right - I need to get off," he said. "See you all tomorrow."

With that, he left, and I turned to mum.

"Right, that's it. Something's definitely going on. Tomorrow night we're going to follow him," I said.

"Oooo...that does sound exciting," said mum. "But what if he sees us?"

"We'll just say we're going for a walk or something. I have to know what he's up to."

It wasn't long after the departure of the star-crossed lovers that the games started.

"I've got a fun game," said Donald, and though I'm usually completely up for late night games, I do like a few drinks inside me first. The prospect of playing silly 'tell all' games with strangers while completely sober was not in the least appealing.

Also, I was starving, and I know you're going to be cross with me for this, but I had a packet of crisps in my bag from the flight and I could fight off the urge to eat them no longer. More than anything in this world I wanted to go back, eat the crisps, have a shower and relax.

I MANAGED to make it back without incident this time, going straight to the right villa. Perhaps it was the lure of the crisps the sent me straight to the right place. I let myself in, rummaged through my bag which was tucked into the far corner of the wardrobe, and pulled out the crisps and a can of coke. Did I not mention that I had coke as well? Oh well, it's only a small can, hardly worth mentioning really.

Then I turned towards the patio doors. It was so hot in the room because mum had turned off the air conditioning when we left. I planned to sit outside in the moonlight and eat the crisps.

But then I saw something amazing...I blinked and checked again. My eyes hadn't mistaken me, there was someone in our pool doing synchronised swimming. It was quite mesmerising. I mean - the lady was really good. She was dressed in a 1950s-style costume and bathing cap and she kept bursting up out of the water, like they do, and kicking her golden legs high into the air while she was upside down. I opened the patio doors and stepped outside, walking as quietly as I could so as not to disturb her.

She didn't stop. She carried on flinging her legs in the air and shooting upwards out of the water with a nose clip on, hair scraped back into a bun, sparkly swimming costume, smiling wildly for an imaginary audience. She didn't see me but I watched her for a while. There was tinny music playing while she performed. She must be a competitive swimmer, she had a proper routine and everything.

"Mary, where are you?" came a voice from behind me. Mum was back. I rushed over to the shrub nearby and stuffed my crisps and coke into it, then ran back towards the villa.

"What are you doing out there?" she asked.

"Come out," I said. "I've just been watching this amazing synchronised swimmer in the pool."

"What?" said mum.

"Come and see," I insisted. "She's really good. She's got a sparkly costume on and everything."

Mum looked at me like I'd gone completely mad, but she followed me outside all the same. When we got there, the swimmer had gone...disappeared into the night with her tape recorder.

I looked at mum and could tell she didn't believe a word I was saying.

"She was here - she had a proper routine and the nose clip and everything, she was really good."

"OK," mum said.

"It's true. She was here."

"Maybe you shouldn't get so much sun tomorrow," she said.

"No, I promise you; I'm not going mad – she was there."

"You must have just seen the moonlight on the water," said mum.

"It wasn't moonlight on water, it was a synchronised swimmer," I insisted, but mum was turning to go back inside.

I'd try to convince her later, once I'd devoured my crisps. Once mum had disappeared into the villa, I rushed over to the shrub and crouched behind it to eat my illicit food. God it was amazing – the crisps tasted so incredibly flavoursome. Too flavoursome in a way - my lips were tingling and my head was buzzing. And the coke made my heart beat furiously. I felt great though. This was wonderful.

Then I heard mum's voice.

Shit.

"What are you doing now?" she asked.

"I'm just looking at this shrub," I said then, in a panic, I tipped the remainder of the crisps into my mouth. Mum had started to walk towards me. There was no way I could finish my mouthful before she got to me, but I didn't want to be caught with a mouthful of crisps. I flapped around, trying to work out what to do. I certainly wasn't going to spit them out – they were way too delicious for that. As mum got close, I freaked. I jumped up, ran to the pool and threw myself into the pool, fully clothed and with so many crisps in my mouth that my face looked like a puffer fish.

"Goodness Mary, I do worry about you," said mum. "I really think you should stay out of the sun as much as possible tomorrow."

I nodded and gave as much of a smile as I could without losing the crisps, and mum went back inside. I finished the crisps, clambered out of the pool and followed her, soaking wet, trying to work out how to explain my actions in such a way she wouldn't try to get me locked up in a lunatic asylum.

SHE FLOATS LIKE A BUTTERFLY AND STINGS LIKE A BEE

"OK everyone, did you enjoy your breakfast?" asked Staff A, smiling and waiting for a response. I sat with my arms folded across my chest and looked around the room. We were a wildly disparate group - different ages, sizes, shapes and backgrounds, but I was fairly confident that we had one thing in common: none of us had enjoyed the Dickensian brown slop that had passed for breakfast. Thank God for the family bag of cheese and onion crisps that I had eaten behind the shrub last night (yes, it was a family bag - don't judge me).

"OK, no huge votes of approval for breakfast then," Staff A continued, having noticed the lack of his response to his enquiry about our food.

"In its favour: it was healthy and it will keep you full, and that's all that really matters. Now then, let's take a quick look at what we're going to be doing today."

I found myself staring at him as he spoke. He seemed to be directing all his comments to Yvonne. Or was that just my imagination? There was definitely a special bond between them. The question was - what bond? The way he'd acted with her at the airport - like long-lost friends...he seemed fascinated by her, but she had insisted she'd never met him before.

"Right," said Staff A, and he held up a blackboard full of activities for the day, detailing what had been arranged for us on the hour, every hour.

"I know it seems like a lot," he said, second-guessing what we were all thinking. "But I urge you to come to everything. As I keep saying, these few days will change your life, but only if you let them. My advice to you is to go with the flow. Stop stressing about not having as much food as you'd like and stop worrying about how hard the exercise will be - just do it. If you're struggling, stop, but don't not start. The worst thing you can do this week is to sit back and not participate. This is week is so short - it'll be gone in no time. If you work hard, you'll lose weight, feel great and have a whole new approach to life."

"That's right," said Staff B, joining 'A' at the front of the room. "I know we keep saying it, but you will get as much out of this week as you allow yourself to. It's day three - in some ways the hardest day. It's the course's 'hump day'. You'll get tired and you'll get hungry and you'll feel really frustrated, but you'll get through it and at the end of the week you'll look back and realise how much you can do if you try your hardest. This will act as inspiration when you get home. Does that make sense to everyone?"

There were murmurs of general agreement because what he said made perfect sense...it just all sounded very hard and I'd rather be lying by the pool eating crisps and watching the late-night synchronised swimmer.

FIRST CLASS of the day was combat skills. Blimey, they like their boxing here. This was the third class in which we'd been asked to don boxing gloves and hit one another. The third one! Luckily, I'd missed the first two. On what planet do you need to do three boxing classes in two days, for God's sake?

We were told to get into pairs and I could see Donald approaching me - there was no way I was going with him. Mum immediately came skipping over to me assuming I'd be with her. This was something I wasn't very keen on at all. She's half my size and I'm half her age. That can't be a fair match-up, surely?

We were given gloves to put on - big, red gloves that you see proper boxers wearing. There was no part of this that seemed OK to me.

"Come on then," said mum, who had been to the two previous boxing classes and clearly thought she knew what she was doing. She danced around like she was Anthony Joshua or something. "Come and get me if you dare," she said.

I held my hands up in the boxing position and copied the stance that Staff B was demonstrating at the front of the class.

"A couple of light punches into your partner's gloves...let's see how you get on," he said.

Mum punched out so ferociously she sent my hands spinning away from my face.

"Gotcha," she said. Christ, she was tougher than she looked.

I shadow boxed back, avoiding hitting her with any force because I knew I'd hurt her.

"Come on, you can do better than that," said mum. "Show us what you're made of."

I continued to tap her gloves with mine and tried to make sure my technique was as good as possible, rather than putting all my power into the shots.

Staff A wandered over. "Is that all you've got?" he asked. "I'm sure you've got more power than that."

I didn't rise to the bait though, I just tapped gently. Then we swapped over again and it was mum's turn to hit. She didn't afford me anything like the same kindness. She whacked me ferociously...with every muscle she had. I swung my arms up to defend myself as the punches rained down on me.

"Now lots of little jabs," said Staff. "Punching as quickly and as hard as you can."

Oh hell. I lifted my arms up to protect myself from the onslaught that was bound to come my way. Mum really swung at me, as I shielded my face from the punches.

When we changed over, I just shadow boxed back.

"Come on, you can do better than that," said mum. "Come on, show us what you're made of."

What happened to the kindly mother who'd knitted me mittens and made me fish fingers for tea? This was a terrible development.

I continued to tap lightly on her gloves, showing admirable restraint while perfecting the noble art. Then Staff A charged over to us. He clearly didn't agree that restraint was a good idea. "I'm sure you've got more power than that."

I didn't rise to the bait, I just tapped gently. "Come on, Mary. The harder you hit, the leaner you'll be." I'm not sure whether this statement would stand up to rigorous scientific examination, but I got what he was saying...put more effort in. But the thing is I didn't want to hit my mum.

When the whistle went and we swapped over again, it was mum's turn to hit. She whacked me ferociously...Blimey. My hands went flying back and mum looked absolutely delighted with herself. Staff A applauded her.

"That's it," he said. "That's the way to do it."

The whistle went and we changed over for the final time. I was completely exhausted...punching was hard, but even standing there with your hands up, being punched, was hard work.

"Now then, come on Mary, you can do it," goaded Staff A, clapping his hands and urging me to put all my weight behind my punches. I swung out a little more than I had previously and, I don't know whether mum wasn't quite concentrating or had dropped her hands a bit, but my fist flew through and caught her right on her left eye with a tremendous thump.

"Ah," she screamed falling to the ground, holding her head. It was like it was all taking place in slow motion...mum spinning backwards, raising her hands to protect her face.

"Oh my goodness, what have you done?" said Staff A, rushing to mum's side, and glaring at me.

"I just did what you told me to do," I said. "In fact, I did what you told me to do when I knew very well that this was exactly what would happen, I should have trusted my own instincts."

I bent down next to mum who was telling me not to worry, and that everything was fine, but I could see her left eye was already starting to close up, and would no doubt go black overnight and leave her looking like she'd been street fighting.

"Let's get you back to the villa," said Staff A, lifting mum gently to her feet, and dropping his arm around her shoulder. I gathered mum's stuff together and ran after them, while the rest of the group stopped and stared at us.

Back at the villa, chef came out of the kitchen with an ice pack and asked what had happened.

"Mary punched her mum in the face," said Staff A.

"It wasn't quite like that," I said. "We were doing the boxing class and I just caught mum on the side of the face."

"Oh my goodness, what on earth made you punch her so hard?"

"I was just doing as I was told," I said. "When I wasn't punching very hard, I was told to hit harder."

"Yes, but not give your mum a black eye!" said Staff A. "No one told you to injure her."

"Are you OK, mum?" I said.

"Honestly, I'm absolutely fine. Please don't worry." But as she looked up at me, her left eye was weeping and already looking swollen, I felt ill to the pit of my stomach.

"You should probably sit this next class out," said Staff A.

"Yes, sure, I think that's a good idea. Thanks," I replied. "I'll go back to my room for a lie down."

"Not you. Your mum," said Staff. "You should do the class; your mum should take it easy."

"Oh yes, of course."

There were two more classes after boxing, the first one to take place on the beach. Mum insisted on coming down with us, but instead of leaping around on the beach, she sat herself down on a rock, and watched as we did what Staff A called "sand training."

In case you were wondering, 'sand training' is when you do lots of activities that are hard enough on solid ground, but you do them on soft sand to make them so much harder.

Mum looked like such a sad, lonely figure, sitting there on the rocks, holding an ice pack to her face, but she insisted that she was OK, and just wanted to watch us. The others in the group had all gone up to her one by one to commiserate with her, and say how awful it was that she got hit in the face. With every comment of support she received, I felt like I was being indirectly castigated for my role in the whole thing.

"OK," said Staff A. "Welcome to "sand training". Can you all line up to face me please."

Staff A was standing with his back to the sea, allowing us to look over at the waves as they crashed down onto the beach while we worked out.

"Let's start with 20 jumping jacks, followed by 20 star jumps, run to Staff B and back, and repeat."

Oh God. This weight loss camp was just about doing the same tortuous exercises over and over again in different environments. Giving the sessions different names like 'sand training' 'hill training' and 'park work out' just allowed the trainers to convince us that we are doing lots of different things.

I was the last one back, of course. They were all running on the spot while they waited for me. I was exhausted already. I looked over at mum, longingly. I wish she'd punched me in the face instead.

Next it was burpees and running with high knees - we did one minute on, 30s off, for six minutes until I thought I might die of exhaustion. The knee lifts meant me whacking my knees into my enormous breasts that bounced around furiously inside my t-shirt even though I was wearing two bras.

After the aerobic exercise was over, I heaved a huge sigh of relief...until he said it was time for press ups, planks, holding squats and leg raises. I was soaking wet, thoroughly exhausted and - oddly - slightly exhilarated. Weird. I hated it, but I loved how it made me feel.

MEETING TRACIE

It was time for lunch. THANK GOD. After we'd eaten, we would be having a talk from a visiting lecturer. The thought of a lecture was quite appealing, and I never imagined I'd be thinking that. But anything that involved sitting down rather than doing star jumps and press-ups was fine by me. And the afternoon activity was a long walk, so at least that shouldn't involve any heart attack-inducing bursts of energy.

Lunch was carrot sticks (I KNOW!!!), with a few pepper and cucumber sticks and a small bowl of homemade hummus.

While we ate, a tall, slim, ferociously heavily-tanned and heavily-made-up woman came in. She must have been mid-50s but was dressed like a young teenage girl, in brightest pink towelling shorts and a white t-shirt with white pom-pom socks inside wedge-heel trainers. Her hair was a bright, artificial blonde - almost white and down to her bottom and her lips were so inflated that they entered the room half an hour before the rest of her. And that's before we got onto the quite extraordinary breasts that looked like they belonged to a woman eight times her size.

It was as if she'd been beamed down from another planet. She looked like Barbie doll's heavily-tanned mum. We all sat there and stared, feeling wildly underdressed in our sweaty old tracksuits.

Staff A jumped up and went over to welcome her. I glanced at Yvonne, by far the most glamorous-looking woman in our midst, and followed her gaze as she took in the woman in front of us. Yvonne's face was an absolute picture. She didn't like this at all. I got the feeling that she didn't like Staff A being so attentive to the new arrival either. I was starting to believe that Staff A and Yvonne really were having an affair.

"OK, can I have your attention?" said Staff A. "I'd like to introduce you to Trace who is going to do a series of short talks about health and fitness issues that you can take back into your everyday lives with you. Tracie, over to you…"

There was a small burst of applause, leading Tracie to bow deeply, and unnecessarily. "Hiya, so I'm Tracie, and as you've been told I'm here to give you a few talks over the next few days, mainly about nutrition and the value of thinking about what you eat and not following fad diets, but also about exercise and why it's so vital that you bring regular movement into your lives."

"This could be hysterical," said mum, adjusting the ice pack on her eye so she could see Tracie properly. "There's no way she's a nutritionist."

"I know," I replied. "This could be really good fun."

We sat back in our seats. Out of the corner of my eye I could see Donald, staring at Tracie like a man possessed. His mouth had dropped open and a little drool had escaped from the side.

"The first thing I'd like to do is address some of the concerns that I know you'll have. Who is this woman before me? What does she know about food? I know I don't look like a nutritionist…I don't look wholesome and well-educated and as if I spend my time growing herbs and making healthy meals. That's because I don't…but I do know all about nutrition and I have lots of ideas for ways in which you can make your diet and your lifestyle healthier without too much effort.

"I was born in England but my mother is French, and when I was

13, we moved to France...people in France have a very difference approach to food, and I will be incorporating some of that thinking into my talks to you over the next few days."

She handed a pile of notes to Simon to hand out and I glanced at Donald who was still staring like some sort of maniac. I felt a pang of anger at his obvious interest in her. I thought he was supposed to fancy me? He was trying to get me to stay in his room one minute, but when a new woman arrived, he was all over her. Not that I was remotely interested, but - you know what it's like - it still smacks a bit when someone goes off you. I'd enjoyed being liked more than I'd realised, perhaps because it was so rare an occurrence.

"Are you OK?" Tracie asked Donald.

"I'm fine," he said, jolting himself out of his reverie and turning to look at the note that Simon had handed to him. "Absolutely fine."

"OK, well as you can see on the sheet, I believe strongly in movement. Not necessarily going to the gym or doing intensive cycling classes - just movement.

"I think one of the first things you need to do if you want to lose weight is to make your days as inefficient as possible. I know that sounds crazy but doing things less efficiently you'll build exercise and movement into your day. So - go the long way round to the bus stop, pace around while you're waiting for the kettle to boil.

"Most people in Europe sit still too much. Research shows clearly that those who move more, even if it's fidgeting or pacing around, are fitter and healthier than those who don't move.

"Let me tell you this - on average, obese people sit for two and a half hours more each day than lean people. In addition, lean people stand and walk for two hours a day more than obese people. How does that make you feel?"

She paused, waiting for someone to answer.

"I feel as if I ought to be fidgeting a bit more," I said. "You know - moving around."

"Yes. No one's saying you have to run a marathon every day or even continue to do the exercise classes that you're doing here today, but try to move more. If you're sitting down to watch tv, get up in the adverts and do a bit of tidying up or walk up and down the stairs a few times. If you've got a pile of three things to take upstairs take them one at a time. If you've got three bags of shopping in the boot - don't do that macho thing of trying to bring them all in at once - bring them in one at a time. Make your life more inefficient."

"This is better than I thought," mum whispered. "Make lots of notes for your blog."

"Oh yes, God - I forgot about the blog," I said, grabbing her pen off her and scribbling notes onto the side of the page. "Remind me every day. I have to start putting posts up as soon as I get back."

"OK, just a few other things to think about," said Tracie, she used her hands a lot when she spoke, displaying fingernails that were about 4" long. Some of them were pierced and had jewels hanging from them. "There are the obvious things that you all know about - park as far away from the place you are going to as possible and walk the final bit, get off the bus a stop earlier, use the stairs rather than the escalators...you know - everyday things that make a real difference.

"Also, why not set the timer on your phone to bleep at 10 to the hour and get up and walk round for 10 minutes, then sit back down and carry on working? It'll make such a difference if you do that as often as you can through the day. Does that make sense?"

She seemed to look directly at me as she said it, so I nodded. It did make sense, to be honest. I knew I was never going to be a gym bunny, or someone who became obsessed with attending exercise classes regularly, but I could easily jump around for 10 minutes every hour. That's what I'd do. Everyone at work would be so impressed...if a little scared.

"OK," said Staff A. "We'll be hearing a lot more from Tracie over the next few days, we just wanted her to introduce herself and give you a range of things you can do at home to continue the good work you've done here. Now then - if anyone wants to take a comfort break, go now, and we'll head off on our three hour walk in 10 minutes. We'll be back in time for dinner."

LEARNING ABOUT WEIGHT LOSS

Mum and I wandered out of the villa onto the beautiful sun-dappled street outside, ready for our huge walk. It would have been so good to lie by the pool with a picnic but - no - more movement was demanded of us.

"What did you think of her?" I asked mum.

"She was better than I expected. I suppose I learnt a few things."

"The main thing I learnt, mum, is that if you have too much filler and too much of a boob lift, you'll look like Barbie."

The two of us cackled, then heard a sound behind us.

"Hello, how did you find my talk?"

Mum and I jumped and spun round to see Tracie standing there. Hopefully she hadn't heard us talking. From the smile on her face it didn't look like it.

"It was great," said mum. "Really good."

"Yes, very useful," I agreed. "Just what we needed."

I noticed she'd changed into proper trainers and was no longer wearing the platform shoes she'd been in earlier. Happily, the bobble socks remained.

"Christ, what happened to you?" she said to mum.

"Oh, that's nothing," said mum. "It's just where Mary hit me."

Tracie looked at me in disbelief, waiting for an explanation.

"I didn't hit her," I said for what felt like the 100th time that day. "I accidentally caught her on the side of her face in a boxing class earlier today. That's all."

"Oh dear. I hope it gets better soon. You'll have a real shiner there," said Tracie, taking my arm and mum's arm and pulling us close. "I want to walk along with you girls."

We followed behind the throng of bodies ahead of us, turning a sharp left to go down the concrete steps onto the beach. It really was a very stunning place... such an open, welcoming beach. As soon as you emerged from the stone stairs, there it was in front of you - the magnificent sea, painted the loveliest blue as if in a van Gogh painting, and miles of sand, fringed with cliffs at the far side. The sky was the colour of dreams - not a cloud in sight, and no sound of anything but the gentle lapping of the water. And, to be fair, the whole place looked much more beautiful when you didn't have to do star jumps and burpee jumps on the sand.

"Come on you lazy buggers, speed up," said Staff A, completely ruining the whole atmosphere.

"Is this what you do full-time?" I asked Tracie. "Going round to these camps lecturing on exercise?"

"I run my own company," she said. "It's health and fitness based, with some personal coaching thrown in. I'm based locally, and work with a number of sports teams and exercise companies."

"Personal coaching - that's exactly what I need," I said. "I just find it so hard not to eat stuff that's bad for me."

"It's not your fault, dear," said mum. "The amount of fat and sugar they put into food these days - it's hard to avoid it. It's really not your fault."

"Oh, but it has to be," said Tracie, stepping over a small sandcastle. "You have to take responsibility, it's the only way."

"How can she take responsibility when manufacturers shove a load of rubbish into food," said mum defensively.

"Don't buy it," replied Tracie. "If a manufacturer sells a product with loads of fat and sugar in it, and you buy it, and get fat. Whose fault is it?"

We walked along without answering her.

"Ultimately, it's your fault," she said. "And if you try to remember that, life will be much easier for you."

"How?" asked mum.

"Because the manufacturers are trying to sell food to you to make a profit. That's their job. That's what they are there for. And they know that the better the food tastes, the more of it people will buy and the more profits they will make. It has to be your job to check whether eating these products is doing you any good or not. We can put pressure on manufacturers to be more honest with us, but at some stage you've got to be honest with yourself, and realise that what they want to achieve and what you want to achieve are polar opposite things. They want you to eat loads of it; you need to stop eating it. How are we going to stop you from eating it?"

Neither me nor mum replied.

"Well, one obvious way is by arming you with all the information you need to make sensible decisions around food. Shall I bore you with some facts and figures, or would you rather me shut up so we can concentrate on walking?"

We were heading up a hill and though I knew there would be magnificent sights when we got up there, it was tough walking and I didn't want to think about it anymore than I had to. "Facts and figures please," I said. These would be useful for my blog posts too.

"OK," she said. "Britain is the fattest country in Europe; it's a problem. But a recent Tory party conference was sponsored by Tate and Lyle. Now, think about that for a minute. If the government is so entranced by money that it can't see the damage that sugar is doing to the population, who's looking out for you? I'll tell you who - you. It has to be you who looks after you: not companies, not the government – you.

"One in three children under 15 is overweight or obese and things are getting worse. Companies are targeting kids from a very young age with sugar, salt and fat. Only you can stop it. Only you can say 'no

- I'm not going to eat that stuff, I'm going to be strong and healthy and eat natural foods that are good for me."

"Yeah," I said. I knew she was right but I was so exhausted I could hardly think, let alone speak. Tracie seemed to be practically skipping up the hill, oblivious to how steep it was. She wasn't remotely out of breath.

"You know what I was saying earlier about doing bits of exercise through the day? Well - you have to do that. YOU. If you don't, you'll get fatter and fatter. Companies are making it as easy as possible for you to access their food.

"Food is being delivered to our doors. Dominoes pizzas and all those lovely big Chinese takeaways - being handed to us on our doorsteps. It's the complete and absolute opposite of how we were meant to consume food. Human beings were designed to go out and hunt for food. You didn't get food without physical exertion first and that was how the body was designed to work.

"Now the most physical thing you have to do is open the door. It just isn't any good for us, you need to try and make yourself walk around, walk to the pizza place at the very least!

"Another interesting fact for you - research shows that the more takeaways there are in an area, the more of it you will eat. It's the same with all addictions, the more readily available alcohol is the more problems people have with drinking. It's a very straightforward thing, but you have to control it. No one else will.

"Avoid takeaways, don't go anywhere near them. Don't tell yourself that you'll just have a healthy dish, keep away from them altogether.

"Think about your body in terms of what it was designed for. It really doesn't want to be crammed full of fatty food and no exercise. It doesn't thrive like that. It won't last a long time like that. Next time you see a really old person, look at what size they are. They'll be thin. Very old people are always thin because fat people die younger. That's how simple and straightforward it is. It's not at all healthy to be fat."

We'd reached the top of the hill where the others were all waiting for us, looking down on the beautiful scenery below. You could see for miles - out to sea where boats were bobbing on the water and right across to the other side of the cliffs. I breathed in the warm air and thought about how there was every chance that I'd die before getting down again. I didn't want to be fat, it wasn't like I was deliberately eating to get fat, I just was fat. It was as much a part of me as my slightly wonky eyebrows or the small scar at the top of my thigh.

"Have you always struggled with your weight?" asked Tracie.

"No - I used to be really thin and really fit. I was a gymnast when I was a girl and trained all the time."

"Oh wow," said Tracie, clearly amazed that there was ever a time when I would dance around in a leotard. "How did you find gymnastics?"

"Quite cruel," I said. "It's a relentless pursuit of perfection. It's a tough sport."

"Yes, the performance sports are," said Tracie with a knowing smile. She'd probably been a dancer or something in her day.

"Portugal's very beautiful, isn't it?" said mum. "I never realised just how lovely it was." She turned to Tracie: "Have you lived here long?"

"No, I was born in England and lived in France when I was a girl," she said. "I didn't come to Portugal until I was in my 20s... chasing a man. An Englishman."

"Ah, that's why you're English is so good," said mum. "I'm always very jealous of people who can speak more than one language."

"You should learn then," said Tracie. "Teach yourself Portuguese, it's very easy."

"I'm too old to learn new things," said mum, sitting down onto the grass, and urging us to join her. Bottles of water were being passed round, so we waited patiently for them to reach us.

"I find I get so tired very easily. Once I turned 65, everything became difficult."

"Are you sleeping OK," asked Tracie. She sat down next to mum and arranged her glossy orange legs in such a way that you could see right up her towelling shorts to where her knickers would have been, if she'd have been wearing any. I noticed with dismay that the orange tan colour didn't stop at the top of her thigh, but continued all the way up.

"No, not really. I just get over-tired, I think. However much I do during the day, I never sleep much. Even on this holiday, Mary's been going to bed before me."

"Sleep's important," said Tracie. "There are lots of things you can do to get a better night sleep. The main thing to start with is a sleep diary, just so you know exactly how much sleep you're getting. Then try going to bed and waking up at roughly the same time each day, that way your body will get used to it, it will fall into a rhythm and you'll fall asleep faster and wake up easier.

"The other thing to do is to swing open the curtains and let the light in first thing in the morning, and take a brisk walk whenever you can. Doing four 30- to 40-minute walks a week helps people with insomnia sleep longer."

"I don't think I can really be bothered," said mum. "I'm OK really, you know."

"Oh no, you must. One large study that followed participants over a 5- to 10-year period found that people who slept less than 7 hours a night were more likely to be obese."

I smiled at her. "Do you have a handy study to quote for every occasion, or do you sometimes make it up?" I said.

"Ha, ha," she said. "I have read lots of studies and I've been giving talks on this subject for 20 odd years. I promise you, I'm not making them up."

We were told to get to our feet and run a little on the spot to get our limbs moving again.

"Shall I give you one tip that will change your life for the better?" said Tracie.

Mum and I looked at one another. "That would be nice," said mum. "Would your advice be - don't ever go to a boxing class with your daughter?"

Tracie smiled. "Maybe that would be a good idea, but my main piece of advice to you, and I suspect this will be more for Mary - make sure you have 60 whole minutes without electronic devices every day.

That's no phone, computer, television - nothing. For an hour. If you do that, you will see your health improve, your mood improve and - eventually - your fitness improve."

"Right," I said. "I can't imagine that."

"No, but you should. You'd be amazed at how your mind calms and your stress recedes. You'll have a whole hour free every day...you could read, have a bath, go for a walk, meditate or do all of them."

"I'll try," I said, but in many ways what she was suggesting would be harder than anything else we'd done. A whole hour? Even at work I didn't go for more than 10 or 15 minutes without a cheeky text from one of my friends, or a sneaky look on Facebook. I'd try though, I just couldn't imagine how successful I'd be.

CHAPTER THIRTEEN: Why do we need to walk so much?

AFTER THE LECTURE FROM TRACIE, I tried not to use my phone for the rest of the walk. I didn't play music or snapchat as I went along, I just enjoyed looking at nature. Blimey, the time dragged. Not because of the nature - the place was beautiful, just because I'm used to walking and talking at the same time as texting and messing around playing games. It felt like the walk went on forever without my phone to distract me.

When we got back, half of us collapsed in the sitting room area of villa one, and the other half decided that enough wasn't quite enough and started swimming in the pool. No need to tell you which half I was in. I lay slumped in the armchair next to mum who looked utterly exhausted. Her eye patch had slipped a little revealing a very red, very closed-up eye beneath it.

"That's the end of your formal exercise for today," said Staff B, standing up before us. "Obviously, if you want to do more, go ahead." He indicated outside, where the bunch of 10 or more nutters were racing up and down the pool. "Tracie's offered to answer any health or fitness questions you may have, but other than that, you're free to go, and I'll see you for our penultimate dinner tonight."

Tracie stood up. "This is nothing formal, but if you do have any questions, I'd be very happy to answer them," she said.

"Why the hell are we doing so much walking?" said a small guy with little round glasses. I'd seen him at some of the classes and he struck me as being very fit. "There seems to be an extraordinary amount of it. I walk every day at home, but just for 40 minutes at a time."

"Good question," I said, nodding enthusiastically.

"OK," said Tracie. "Well - it's a good way to see the place. Obviously, we're in a lovely part of the world...many of you haven't been here before and won't come here again, so it's good to take time out to look around and see things. But in terms of fitness, the answer is very simple - the reason we walk so much is because walking is exceptionally good for you."

"I bet she's got a study that proves it," I whispered to mum.

"Let me prove this to you," said Tracie, and mum and I did a secret high five. "Let me prove to you that walking can save your lives."

"Save our lives?"

"Yep," she said. "Does anyone know why?"

"Because you get your heart rate going, and your limbs moving?" I ventured.

"Star pupil. Well done," said Staff B, moving to stand next to Tracie. Staff B was quite pale, and when he stood next to her it threw into stark relief just how orange she was.

I looked up to catch mum's eye but she was looking through the patio windows, watching the seagulls dance elegantly through the sky over the pool, straining to watch them with her one good eye.

"Sorry to interrupt you Tracie, but we forgot to give out your snacks earlier, so I'll hand them out to you now, while you're listening," said Staff B.

"Oh My God - that's the greatest news ever," I blurted out, rather too loudly, encouraging titters of laughter from those assembled. It suddenly dawned on me that the group here were the rebels of the course, the kids on the back seat of the bus, the ones flicking bits of paper at the teacher. The well-behaved kids were outside doing extra homework.

It was quite a jolly moment.

Then I was handed half an apple. HALF AN APPLE! And my mood bombed.

"Since I'm a star pupil, can I have a whole apple?" I tried.

"Nope."

Blimey these people didn't know the meaning of the word 'snack' they should see me hoovering nachos while watching Netflix.

"OK, the importance of walking," continued Tracie. She had turned down her half of an apple. She said she didn't want to ruin her dinner. "I need to start by telling you a story...a story about bus drivers and bus conductors."

This wasn't the most promising of starts to a story, but I decided to bear with it.

"In 1949, Jerry Morris, a professor of social medicine in London, conducted a study to compare the rates of heart disease between London bus drivers and conductors. "The drivers and conductors were from similar social backgrounds; however, there was a marked difference in the rates of illness between them.

"Morris's study showed that conductors were half as likely to die from a heart attack as drivers. He wanted to know why. In the end, he concluded that it was because in every working day, while drivers were typically sedentary, conductors walked all day.

"So, it was more than 50 years ago that doctors realised that regular exercise through the day was a life saver."

"Gosh, is that right? That's really interesting," said Simon.

"Yes - it's very interesting because the difference between the drivers and the conductors and their life expectancies was so stark. Back then there were just two people working on every bus - a driver who sat in his seat all day and drove, and a conductor who scrambled around - up and down the stairs, making his way among passengers, and collecting fares at every stop.

"Seeing the results and working out why, was one of the first times that doctors began to appreciate the link between early death and an inactive, sedentary life. Being overweight or obese wasn't taken much into account back then as most people were of normal weight. The drivers in the study weren't any more or less overweight than the conductors. Now, a half century later, the link between a sedentary life and early death has been reconfirmed in dozens of studies worldwide.

"Exercise is important...not just for weight loss or toning or anything like that, but for living. If you want to live a long and healthy life, exercise has to be a cornerstone of that. Walking is excellent exercise. That's why we do so much of it on the course."

She paused at this stage, as if giving us all time to take in the magnitude of what she was saying. A silence fell over us. I'd definitely try and walk more when I got back. I could easily get off the bus early or something...be more like the conductor than the driver.

"Any more questions?" she asked.

I had one. I always have questions: "You said when we were talking before that manufacturers were putting loads of sugar in our foods and we needed to make sure we didn't buy it. Why do they do that? Surely if they just made food healthier, a lot of the western world's problems would go away?"

"Yes, but their priority isn't trying to solve the problems of the western world. You are talking about commercial companies, trying to make money, and they sell more food if it's laced with sugar and fats. The reason that didn't happen in the past is because we have different tastes today.

"The reason for this? And one of the big problems of modern living? Freezers. Yep. More than 95% of people have freezers in the UK, and much of the food that we put in the freezer has to be highly processed in order for it to survive the process. Doing this removes flavour, so then you have to add in more sugar, salt and fat to get the flavour back and make them taste nice again. In the past people just ate fresh food and bought fresh every day, because they didn't have freezers so they had to. We were much healthier without them. The healthiest way to live is to buy fresh food every day."

Again, she paused, and I looked at mum who was trying to fix her eye-patch. Simon leaned over as if to lend a hand, but I batted him away before he could help. "I've got this, thanks," I snarled, as he retreated.

"Everything OK?" asked Tracie.

"Oh yes, completely fine," said mum. "I'm really enjoying listening to you. Do carry on."

"OK - well, just one final point about processing food is that it makes the food easier for the body to digest. Do you remember what I was saying earlier about making life as difficult for yourself as possible? Making yourself use energy whenever you can? Well, the same applies here - normally you have to use energy to break up the food that you eat. The body has to break up the various components and work hard to digest it, and a certain percentage of the calorific contact of the food is used up doing this.

"But if all the work has been done for you in the processing, then all the calories in the product go straight into your body without you expending any of them in breaking it down, so food is more calorific as a result.

"You need to eat healthy, unprocessed food whenever you can."

"What? Never use the freezer?"

"I don't have one. I don't think they're a good idea," said Tracie. "But if you've got a large family and rely on them, the tip is just to make sure you eat fresh, healthy, unprocessed food as much as you can, and only use the freezer for emergencies.

There was a lot of mumbling at this...a lot of displeasure at the thought of not being able to pull burgers out of the freezer and shove them straight into the oven at tea-time.

"Any more tips?" asked Donald.

"I think that's about it for now," she said. "There will be more time to talk tomorrow."

"OK, so there's nothing else you do to keep yourself looking so fit and...if you don't mind me saying...amazing, that we should be doing?"

"Oh goodness, thank you," said Tracie, blushing a little through her radiant orange skin. "I do take a low dose aspirin daily. That's not a bad idea as you get older. It's controversial, I know, and I wouldn't advise taking drugs for the sake of it, but a blood thinning medicine like aspirin helps to prevent heart attacks and strokes. My sister had a stroke a few years ago, and I was classified as high risk, so I take one every day. Aspirin makes the blood less sticky and helps to prevent heart attacks and strokes. One with breakfast dramatically reduces the risks."

BUM FLASHING

Dinner on the penultimate evening was slightly better (but we're coming from quite a low point). Instead of the usual bowl of indescribably bad soup, we had salmon with broccoli and even a yoghurty thing for dessert which tasted quite sweet and delicious. It was served in a tiny bowl the size of an egg cup, of course, so when I'd eaten it, I ran my finger round the inside of the bowl, trying to get every last morsel out. Then I tried to put my tongue into it to make sure there was nothing left, but mum took it off me and told me to behave.

After dinner, there was the usual bee-line for the sofas and the commencement of the games. It was like living in the past, in the days before televisions. But none of that bothered me because I was entertaining myself by watching Yvonne and, as always, she got to her feet and said that she was leaving for the spa down the road.

I looked at mum. I wasn't sure whether she'd want to come on this expedition with me, given how exhausted she looked, and given that her eye was now completely closed up and a rather unattractive shade of grey. But I thought I'd try anyway.

"Come on, Yvonne's gone - let's sneak out and follow her. I'm dying to know where she goes," I said, nudging her.

"Wouldn't it be nicer to sit here and drink herbal tea with the others?" she replied.

"No," I replied, honestly. "Why would you want to do that when you could be launching yourself into the night on an extraordinary expedition."

"Really?" said mum. "An 'extraordinary expedition' to see whether Yvonne is meeting up with Staff A? Good job you don't work for the secret service, you'd be blown away by the things they have to do."

"Are you coming or not?" I said, not dignifying her comment with an answer.

"Okay," she said wearily. "But only so I'm there to keep an eye on you if anything goes wrong."

"Fair enough," I said. "I wish I had camouflage gear with me, and a head torch."

"Oh God," said mum. "Let's go."

We left the villa, claiming tiredness and said we were heading off to get an early night, but turned left at the top on the street, and took the road to the stone steps which led down onto the beach, rather than back to our villa.

"How do we know where to go?" asked mum. "We can't go to every bar in town."

"I don't think there are many bars," I replied. I did a recce by talking to Abi and she said there were three cafes and a hotel. The hotel is where the gym and spa are, and where Yvonne claims she goes. Let's start there."

"OK," said mum. "But I can't go in like this, can you put my patch back on my eye for me. I'll scare everyone."

I helped mum to apply the cotton pad and large plaster, and we continued on our way.

"I'm going to have a glass of wine tonight," I said. "Just a small one."

"Really? What, and undo all the good work? Why don't you just have a glass of water like I'm going to."

"Because I really want a glass of wine. Come on I've been so good all the way through - I haven't had any sneaked in snacks or anything..." (ssshhhhh....no need to mention the three packets of crisps - mum doesn't need to know).

"OK, but just have a small one," said mum. We walked along the beach towards the seafront cafes, and I scanned the area as we went - looking out for Yvonne and Staff A. I didn't even know whether Staff had followed her this time because he hadn't been in dinner tonight, but I suspected he had. I peered out, watching for every movement. I felt like a fugitive avoiding arrest.

"There it is," I said, pointing to a large hotel which looked as if it had lovely views of the sea. It was very plush. I imagined that it would probably have a very nice spa.

"What are you going to do?" asked mum.

"Well, why don't we go in and see whether they are in the bar?"

"OK," said mum. "Of course, Yvonne could be in the spa and Staff A could be in his room doing press ups or something."

"Yes, I realise that," I said. "But unless we go and check things out, we'll never know."

"We should look in the spa first," said mum. She'd obviously worked out that any investigation headed up by me would attempt to start in the bar.

"Or the main bar," I tried. "We could have a quick drink while making a plan?"

"No - spa first. That's where she said she was going so we should check that out. Then, if she's not there, we'll know she lied and can try and find her."

"OK," I said, quite impressed that mum had thought this through so carefully.

First, we walked into the gym, and pretended we were hotel guests taking a look round. There was no sign of either Yvonne or Staff A in there. It was a nice place. Very plush, with lots of equipment, screens flashing on every machine and music sweeping through the place.

There weren't many people there, and those who were there didn't seem to be doing a great deal, it was more the sort of gym you were seen in rather than one you worked out in.

"OK, she's not here," I said to mum, stating the bleeding obvious. "Let's check out the spa area."

So, we walked out of the gym and into the spacious, pine changing room - it looked and smelled like a giant sauna. There were steam rooms, jacuzzi, saunas and 'splash pool' leading off the main changing room - each one was behind a door. There was a big pile of fluffy towels outside each of the doors.

"You'll have to get undressed, you can't walk into the steam room like that," said mum, flicking her hand to illustrate my inappropriate clothing.

"Damn," I muttered. This was all getting to be quite hard work.

I slipped off my leggings and t-shirt and went to wrap one of the lovely soft, fluffy towels around me. Of course, it was far too small and didn't come near to covering me. I grabbed another one and tried to arrange the two of them so that I wouldn't expose myself to everyone in the steam room. Then I went in. The place was full of steam - which, I guess, is what I was expecting, but I hadn't thought through the fact that I wouldn't be able to see anyone in there. I sat down and waited for my eyes to adjust. There was just one woman in there. Considerably older than Yvonne. On to the next room. The sauna was easier to see in - three women, no Yvonne. Then I walked into the room marked splash pool.

"I'll come with you," said mum. "I can go in here in my clothes." She followed me through the door which led to two small swimming pools. The glass roof had been opened so it was like being outside. There were about 20 people there - some swimming but most of them lounging on sunbeds and reading or talking. Clutching my towels tightly, I walked around, checking each face in turn to see whether Yvonne was there. No. No sign of her. So, I walked back to the door, reaching to push it open so we could go back into the changing room. But reaching out for the door involved letting go of my towel, before I could stop it, the first towel had fallen to the ground, quickly followed by the second one.

Oh God.

My rather large bottom was exposed to all of the splash pool users in the lovely Portuguese spa.

"Put it away, Mary," mum said, under her breath.

WHEN MOUTH-TO-MOUTH GOES WRONG

I got changed as quickly as possible and tried to forget about the fact that everyone in the spa had seen my bum.

"They weren't looking. No one noticed," mum kept saying, in an effort to reassure me. But I'd seen the looks of horror and heard the gasps as my towel hit the floor.

"I'll definitely need a glass of wine now," I said, as we walked into the hotel bar.

"I thought that might be the case," said mum.

I didn't loiter when we entered the bar. I walked straight up and ordered a large glass of wine for me and sparkling water for mum, then took a massive swig out of it and almost reeled from the power of the taste. I'd drunk nothing but water and three cans of coke since I arrived in the country. The taste of wine almost knocked me off my feet.

"Gosh, these small glasses are big, aren't they?" I said to mum, indicating the size of my large glass. "I'm glad I didn't have a large one."

"Golly, yes," said mum. "There's no way you'll be able to drink all that."

Does she know nothing about me at all?

"Come on - let's take a wander and see whether we can find them.

I know you won't relax until you've seen them," said mum, taking a delicate sip out of her glass

We walked around, cautiously looking for Staff A and Yvonne. In my head, the plan was for us to see them, but for them not to see us. I hadn't quite worked out how we were going to do this. I realised it would probably involve me throwing myself behind a pillar or a pot plant.

We walked around a couple of times, looking into all the nooks and crannies. I even went into the ladies to check, and stood for an unseemingly long time outside the gents.

Nope. They weren't there.

"We'll drink these then go to the other little bars on the beachfront," I said. "If they're not in any of those, then they are not in town tonight."

Mum smiled and shook her head at me. I know she thought I was mad, but it was quite intriguing the way they sneaked out like that. And I didn't believe that they'd never met before this holiday, the way he reacted to her at the airport was straight out of Love Story.

We took our glasses over to a table near to the window. All of the tables around us were full of people chatting in groups, enjoying food and drink. There were bowls of fries, oven baked brie and piles of chicken wings on the table next to me. I was dying to reach over and take one, but I managed to control myself.

I just watched them instead. Staring at the woman as she put a potato skin, loaded with cheese and bacon into her mouth.

"Stop looking like that," said mum.

"I can't help it." I replied. "It's torture sitting here next to them."

The woman eating the potato skin was English, as was everyone else in the group. They chatted about people they knew from home and what they were up to. And I relaxed as the familiar sounds of people discussing Love Island and Brexit washed over me. I was starting to really enjoy my evening away from the camp.

Then, suddenly, the women I'd been studying started having a coughing fit. She fell to the ground in a dramatic fashion, holding her chest. She looked in considerable pain, but no one at her table did anything, they just looked around at each other. The woman writhed on the floor - reaching up to them, as if to indicate that she needed help.

I'd done a first aid course a few years ago, so fancied my chances of keeping her heart going until the ambulance came. I jumped out of my seat and ran over to her, aggressively turning her onto her side and opening her airway to check whether she was breathing. I tipped her neck back and prepared to give her mouth-to-mouth.

"Call an ambulance," I shouted to mum.

I felt amazing. Invincible. I was Wonder Woman. I'd be in every national newspaper and probably on that morning TV show with Piers Morgan. I'd definitely go to Downing Street and meet the Prime Minister.

I leaned in to give the woman mouth-to-mouth and save her from certain death when she suddenly pushed me away dramatically. She used quite a lot of force for a woman who'd been at death's door two minutes ago. Then she sat up and wagged her finger at me: "What are you doing? Get off me."

"I thought you were having a heart attack or something. I was trying to help," I said. I was alarmed and confused at the odd reaction that my kind act had provoked.

"We're playing a murder mystery game and you're completely ruining it."

"Oh sorry," I said. "I thought you were in trouble."

"No. We picked names out of a hat earlier and I'm the victim. I have to die. It's part of the game"

"Oh, I see. I'm sorry," I repeated, as a couple more people joined their table.

"Oh, my goodness," said one of them. "That's the flasher from the spa."

Everyone on the table was now staring at us. Mum looked completely baffled. I don't think she knew what was going on.

"Come on, we're going," I said. Mum stood up and the two of us spun round and walked dramatically away from the table...just as Staff A and Yvonne walked through the door.

"Hit the floor!" I shouted to mum, as if a gun-wielding terrorist had just entered the building. We both fell to our knees and crawled back under the table of the group whose game I'd just wrecked.

"What the hell is she up to now?! I heard one of them say.

Staff and Yvonne walked to the bar.

"Quick, let's go," I said to mum, and the two of us speed crawled to the exit, darted out and ran down the road, not stopping until we reached the beach.

"God that was fun," I said to mum.

"No, that was ridiculous. Everyone in there thinks we're insane."

"But at least we know that they are definitely having an affair," I said to mum.

"Unless they are just friends?" she suggested.

"But then why would they sneak out, and why would she lie about where she was going?"

Mum shrugged, as we walked back over the sand towards the stone steps. "It's odd, isn't it? You just wouldn't have put those two together - they seem such different people."

"I know. I think that's what's so intriguing. I bet he flew her out here specially to see her. I'm glad we came down to find out. And thanks for coming with me," I said. "It would have been horrible if I'd gone by myself."

"No problem my little flasher," she said, laughing as she said it. "Honestly, you should have seen their faces when your towel dropped. They were a picture."

"I thought you said no one saw..."

"Ah, yes - I lied about that. They all saw," she said. And we both burst out laughing.

MY LEGS WERE REALLY ACHING by the time I got back to the villa. It had been an action-packed evening: flashing, ruining a party game, then crawling out of the pub on hands and knees.

"Why do the oddest things always happen to me?" I asked mum, forlornly. "Other people manage to go through days without punching their mother in the face or anything. I wish I could be like other people. Did they really see my bottom in the sauna? That's so embarrassing."

Mum burst into laughter, and before long I was laughing too. "It really was the most ridiculous evening, wasn't it?" she said through spluttering laughter, as she gave me a hug and sat down on the bed next to me. "Honestly..."

Then she gasped and pointed outside. Her mouth was wide open. I followed her finger and there - in our pool again - was the synchronised swimmer. She danced merrily through the water while the two of us sat on my bed watching her.

"She's really good, isn't she?" I said.

"Yes," said mum. "She's wonderful. I thought you'd lost your mind, talking about women dancing in the pool. But look at her - she's there and she's really good. Let's go and watch her from the poolside."

Mum undid the back door and the two of us walked onto the patio. The same music was playing as last time I'd seen her - gently drifting through the night air as she danced around. She pushed herself up out of the water effortlessly as we walked towards the pool, but as we got close the same thing happened...she saw up and swam towards the edge, leapt up onto the side with considerable agility, and ran away, tearing off her sparkly swimming hat to reveal a streak of blonde hair, grabbing her music player and disappearing into the trees.

"Oh, that's such a shame," said mum, looking really disappointed. "I wanted to watch her."

"I know, mum. Me too. Oh, hang on. She's dropped something," I walked to the edge of the pool and there lay her swimming hat...it was very old-fashioned with small flowers on it, and not sparkly at all. It must have been the reflections of the moonlight off the water catching it as she danced that had made it look as if it was covered in sequins.

I carried the hat back to where mum was waiting. Inside the cap, the initials NSF/TM were sewn.

"I need to take it back to her," I said to mum.

"Well, leave it here - she's bound to come back when she realises she left without it."

"No - I mean I want to find her - I want to know about her."

"Oh God," said mum, seeing the excitement burning in my eyes. "We don't have time for more spying missions. When are you going to go off and find her? Tomorrow is the last day."

"I'll go in the morning," I said. "I'm not doing boxing and combat training for three hours, that's for sure. I'm lethal."

"You're not lethal," said mum.

"Really? Have you looked in the mirror recently?"

Mum shook her head and climbed into bed. "I'm just thrilled that a synchronised swimmer really exists and you're not barking mad."

I lay back on my bed, still holding the cap, my mind spinning with thoughts and plans about how I might find the mystery swimmer.

As I lay there in the darkness, unbeknownst to me, the lady came back and, silently, while mum and I slept, she scoured the garden looking for her cap. She looked through the shrubs and moved the sunbeds and deck-chairs around, but it was nowhere to be found. Disappointed, she left, off into the night from whence she came

IN SEARCH OF THE PHANTOM SYNCHRONISED SWIMMER

I woke up the next morning for our final full day in camp still holding onto the swimming cap. It took me a few moments to remember what the odd item in my hand was. I had clutched it all night, leaving my palm sweaty underneath its rubbery skin. I felt a wave of excitement when I saw it, and shot out of bed still gripping onto it. Today was the day when I would find synchro woman.

I went over to where my phone was plugged into the wall, near the dressing table on the other side of the room and typed in Google to begin investigating. It was only 5am - earlier than I'd been up all week. It came as no surprise to me at all that when there was the prospect of physical exercise, I had absolutely no desire to get out of bed; but when there was a mysterious synchronised swimmer to locate I was out of bed faster than you could say 'nose clip'.

Mum slept soundly beside me while I put the initials embroidered into the cap into Google, hoping that the letters would mean something; that they would reveal where the swimmer had come from. NSF/TM: the letters had to be the name of a swimming club or something.

But...Nope. Nothing. Next, I googled synchronised swimming

clubs in the area but I couldn't find anything. This sleepy region of Portugal was not awash with sporting amenities, certainly not of the water dancing kind, but synchro woman must be based locally, surely. I couldn't believe the woman came miles to use my pool. That made no sense at all.

There was a sports centre with a swimming pool in the area and it seemed to be a short bus ride away, so I figured that would probably be my first stop. There must be someone there who could tell me where synchronised swimming classes were held in the area. They might even be listed on the sports centre's website but it was impossible to tell by looking at it because it was all in Portuguese; no English at all.

I worked out that I could get the bus from outside the beachfront cafes. It was only a few stops.

As I studied the bus route, I heard a small movement behind me as mum woke up. "Goodness, what are you doing up so early?" she asked.

"Trying to work out how to find the synchronised swimmer," I said.

"Mind if I put the light on?".

"Of course not. I was only sitting in the dark so I didn't wake you."

Mum switched on the light by her bed and I looked over at her.

"Oh. My. God," I screamed. "Oh Christ."

"What?" Mum looked perplexed.

"Your eye!" I said. "It looks like you've been in a fight with Mike Tyson...and lost."

Her eye was black and completely sealed up. It was puffy and tender looking. It really did look like a boxer's eye the day after a fight.

"Oh, then it must look worse than it feels," said mum. "It actually it's a lot less painful today than it was yesterday."

"I think you need to see a doctor," I said. "Do you want to come with me today on a hunt for Synchro Woman and we'll find a doctor?"

"I'm sure there's no need," said mum. "And if this is your way of co-opting me into a chase around the country looking for someone whose face we've never seen and whose name we don't know, you can forget it."

"No, I'm being serious mum," I said (and I was). "I'll forget the hunt for the synchronised swimmer - we'll just go and get you to a doctor. We should have gone yesterday. Honestly, it looks really bad."

"But surely the people on the course would have suggested a doctor if they thought I needed one."

"Yeah, you'd think so," I said. "But they're all army people, you could probably lose a leg and they'd get you to hop through the exercises. They don't do 'injuries'."

"I suppose so," she said. "But it doesn't feel too bad at all. I'm sure in a couple of days it'll be perfect."

"But what if it's not? What if it's infected and you lose an eye and have to walk around wearing an eye patch for the rest of your life? Won't you wish you'd been to see a doctor then?"

"Yes, I suppose," she said. "And I can't really do three hours of combat training this morning anyway, can I? Let's go and find a doctor."

"Good, I'll see if google knows where the nearest one is," I said.

"And I suppose we might as well make some initial enquiries about the synchronised swimmer while we're out and about. I know how keen you are."

"Oh good," I said, rubbing my hands together in glee as I got ready. "I'm SO keen. You have no idea. This'll be fun. I know where the local sports centre is, and how to get there, I think we should start there in our hunt, but only when I've worked out where the nearest doctor's surgery is."

We walked the now familiar path and headed down the stone steps and across the beach to find the bus that would take us to the local sports centre.

I had googled medical centres and discovered that next to the pool complex was a parade of shops in which there appeared to be both a doctor's surgery and a pharmacy. It struck us that if we went into the chemist shop first and talked to the pharmacist, he or she could advise as to whether we should see a doctor. The pharmacist might even be able to advise as to the best way to get an appointment.

The bus journey was extremely short - just a couple of stops - it took about 10 minutes to get there and both mum and I looked at one another knowingly. We should have walked it. "What have they been saying to us all week?" said mum. "Walk whenever you can."

"Yes, I agree," I said. "We'll walk back."

My excitement about finding the synchro woman had by now mounted to such fever pitch that I would have promised to walk to the moon and back. I was ready to go inside and begin the search. I had the hat tucked into my handbag and mum by my side, looking like a pirate in her large, homemade eyepatch. What could possibly go wrong?

We queued up and waited patiently at the main reception with all the children clutching their towels as they bought tickets for a morning swim.

"I wish I spoke Portuguese," I said to mum. "Even just a few words would make it easier. I don't know how I'm going to explain to this woman what I'm after."

"I was thinking the same thing myself," said Mum. "If she only speaks a few words of English, "synchronised" is unlikely to be one of them."

Once we reached the front of the line, excitement had turned to panic as I realised I was going to have to explain my desires to this woman and there was no doubt that I was going to sound very odd.

"Synchronised swimming," I said, waving the hat around. "Is there anyone here who I can talk to about synchronised swimming?"

The woman looked at me blankly.

"Synchronised swimming," I repeated, as if that was going to help in anyway. Then, the inevitable happened.

"Show me," she said.

"OK," I replied, and began leaping around in the reception in my best interpretation of a synchronised swimmer. I had the fixed smile, the sudden upward jumps and even a few high kicks in order to convey my message. The entire row of children, and most of the people in the café opposite were watching, intrigued by my sudden performance.

Remarkably, the woman on reception seem to understand me.

"Ah," she said. She looked again at the hat and a look of genuine comprehension passed over her face.

"I am understanding now. Down to end on the left. Is there."

"Who is there?" I asked.

"Person of the hat."

"The person who owns this hat is here?" I said. I couldn't believe it. I'd hoped they'd be able to translate the letters on the hat for me, or advise me where to go next, I never expected to be directed straight to Synchro Woman's office.

"Come on," I said. "We're in business."

"Wonderful!" said mum. "And really astonishing that she knew what you wanted from that little routine in reception."

"Cheeky," I said. "That was a magnificent display of floor synchronised swimming, even if I say so myself."

We walked towards the room that we had been directed to by the lady on reception, when we passed a ladies toilet and mum said she had to go.

"Really? Can you not wait?"

"I'll be two minutes," she insisted

I waited patiently for way more time than is necessary for someone to go to the loo. I had no idea what on earth she was doing in there. I just wanted to go and find the synchronised swimmer. So, I walked down to the room to which the lady had suggested we go, and knocked gently on the door. There was no answer.

"Hello, is anyone there," I said.

I turned the handle cautiously and the door opened onto a small room that looked as if it had been set up for fitness testing. There were scales, callipers and measuring tapes. I slammed the door shut quickly. I didn't need to see callipers and weighing scales. Urgh. It was like a torture chamber in there.

"There you are!" said mum, who had emerged from the ladies

toilet and was wandering down the corridor with a familiar-looking woman.

"Look who I found in the ladies," said mum, indicating Tracie standing beside her.

"Hi, how are you doing?" I said. "Have you heard about our mission?"

"Indeed I have," said Tracie. "And I'm going to accompany you. I know exactly where you need to go, follow me..."

And so, the three of us walked confidently through the sports centre, me waddling along, Tracie striding confidently ahead, orange skin gleaming in the sunshine, and mum shuffling along. pirate-style. beside us.

"In here," said Tracie, indicating a door that was nowhere near the one that the receptionist had told us to go to. She knocked gently on it but there was no answer, then she knocked again.

I'll just peek in," she said, turning the handle, but the door wouldn't open.

"Damn, it's locked."

All three of us stood there looking at the locked door for a little while until she had a brainwave.

"I know," she said. She marched off again with the two of us running along behind her, and spoke to a small, tubby woman in Portuguese.

"Follow," said the woman, leading the way through the sports centre. She had an oddly wide gait for someone so small and as she walked, she had her hands resting on her hips. She looked like a cowboy who'd just got off his horse.

"She knows where to go," said Tracie. So, we followed John Wayne through the centre, still in search of the owner of a rather fancy synchronised swimming cap.

The woman led us to an office right back at the back of the building.

"Thank you so much," I said, as she opened the door and talked to a very tall man inside. They had quite a conversation before he said.

"I take you."

So now there were five of us on our mission, walking round the building. The very tall man, the small, fat woman who walked like a cowboy, mum looking like a pirate, me waddling along to keep up, and Tracie with her bright orange, Day-Glo legs.

He took us to another room but that was empty too. Where on earth was this synchro woman? Unfeasibly tall man spoke to Day-Glo legs woman, while cowboy lady watched and nodded. Pirate and I just looked on forlornly. There was lots of shrugging and raised voices.

"No one knows," Tracie said eventually.

"OK," I said, a little confused. "The lady on reception said it was that room at the end of the corridor, right where you come into the centre."

"Oh," said Tracie. "Right - let's go back there then."

So, back we all trouped, through the sports centre, dropping off the man and woman who had accompanied us (but been no use at all), as we went. Then we followed the corridor back and I said: "There, that's the room the lady on reception said was the right one."

"No - that's not right. That's my room."

"Your room? So, you work here?"

"Yes - I do the fitness and nutrition for the squads here."

"Oh. How odd."

"Look, don't worry. We'll find a first aid person somewhere," said Tracie. "They are probably just busy treating someone."

"No - we're not after a medic," I said.

"Yes - for your mother's eye," said Tracie. "I thought that's what you had come for - to find a medical specialist."

"Oh, no, that's my fault," said mum. "I must have confused you when you asked about my eye and I said we were going to find a doctor. We're actually at the sports centre on a rather more complicated mission."

"We are here to ask about synchronised swimming. I found this cap," I said, pulling the swimming hat from my bag.

Tracie practically swooned in front of us and leant heavily against the wall. "Where did you find that?" she said, her eyes wide with excitement.

"It was left by our pool," I said.

"That was your pool?"

"Yes, a lady has been doing synchronised swimming in the pool outside our villa. She left this hat and I wanted to return it to her."

"That's me," said Tracie. "That's my hat."

"It's YOU," both mum and I declared. "Why did you run away when you saw us?"

"I didn't know it was you. I thought you were coming to tell me to get out of your pool, so I got out before you could tell me off."

"We were coming to watch you...you were brilliant."

"Oh," said Tracie, all smiles. "Thank you. That's so sweet."

"How did you learn to do that?"

"It's a long story," said Tracie. "Shall we get some herbal tea?"

"That would be great," I said, hoping I could order a sneaky cappuccino instead. "But first let's go to the pharmacy to get mum sorted, then I want to hear all about this."

LEARNING THE TRUTH ABOUT NSF/TM

The three of us went to the pharmacy around the corner from the sports centre where a very friendly pharmacist said he thought mum's eye was best left alone. He recommended painkillers and some antibacterial eye drops to keep it all as clean as possible, and told her to visit her own GP back in England if it hadn't improved over the next couple of days. He also sold her an eye patch, much to my joy, and recommended regular ice packs and getting lots of rest. Mum nodded gratefully and bought the drugs he advised.

Then it was time to hear Tracie's story.

"I was a very talented synchronised swimmer when I was younger," she said, as we sat sipping some revolting green tea in the cafe near the sports centre (no luck with my attempts to order cappuccino). "I competed for France, then in 1987 I was selected for the World Cup, held in Egypt."

"Oh, my goodness," said mum. "That's amazing. You must be really good."

"I was very good," said Tracie. "But I struggled with terrible stage fright, and I was never very good in the big tournaments. I just froze. That's what I did in the World Cup...I panicked and I fell out of synchro. We were on for medal, and could have won gold, but I messed up and we dropped out of the medals, we came fourth.

"That's the worst place to come...to just miss out on a medal. It was awful. And it was all my fault."

"Oh no," said mum, "I'm sure it wasn't all your fault. It can't have been."

"Yep," said Tracie, nodding vigorously. "All my fault. I did a completely different routine to the others - I just forgot everything."

"You shouldn't beat yourself up," I said, though I did make a mental note to try and find a video of that World Cup - Tracie doing a completely different routine to the rest of the team sounded hysterical. "Fourth in the World Cup is brilliant. The World Cup is probably like the Olympics of synchronised swimming. That's brilliant."

"Yes," mum said. "Really brilliant. Well done."

"Well, it's strange you should mention the Olympics, because they took place the next year," said Tracie, looking even more mournful. "And I was selected. I couldn't believe it. I had another chance."

"Oh, that's fantastic," I said. "I love a story with a happy ending."

"Yeah, except that when I got there, I was so nervous. It was in Seoul and I'd never been anywhere like that before. I was just terrified...and I did exactly the same thing again...I messed up and France missed out on the medals. We came fourth. Again."

"Oh dear, I'm so sorry," said mum. "Really, though - you shouldn't blame yourself. It's quite natural to be nervous performing in front of all those people."

"You're very kind, but it was awful. I stopped the sport as soon as I got back to France and I never did any synchro again...until about two weeks ago. The guys at the sports centre found out about my background and were keen for me to start running synchronised swimmer classes. I froze when they first asked me and said there's no way I could do it, but Rodrigo - the guy in charge here - told me to think about it...and the more I thought about it, the more I thought that I'd actually quite like to do that. But I didn't know whether I could remember anything, so when I came to the camp to give the talks, and saw all those empty pools, I thought I'd come back at night time and have a practice while you were all having dinner. I didn't want to ask anyone in case it drew attention to me. I just wanted a bit of time in the pool by myself to check whether I was still comfortable in the water."

"You certainly looked it," said mum. "You were really impressive when we saw you."

"Thank you," said Tracie. "I loved it. I loved every minute of it, and I'm definitely going to teach lessons at the swimming pool and try and build up a young squad."

"That's amazing," said mum. "I'm so pleased. And I'm sorry if we scared you off when you were practising - we didn't mean any harm at all - we just wanted to watch because you were so good."

I handed the swimming cap over. "Sounds like you're going to need this," I said. "Just one more question - what do the letters inscribed on the inside mean?"

"Oh - they are from my international days - so synchronised swimming in French is nage synchronisée and the 'f' is for France because that's who I was competing for. My name is Tracie Molton, so: NSF/TM is the national team and the swimmer."

"Got it," I said.

Despite mum and I saying that we would walk back, in the end we got a cab with Tracie. She was coming over to join us all for our last evening in camp. We sat comfortably on the back seat and watched the beautiful scenery rush past us.

"That thing in the sports centre was quite funny when you think about it," I said. "You and two senior members of staff in there all joining in the hunt for you."

Tracie smiled. "Yes, that is very funny. I was just asking everyone where the first aid person was."

"I'll miss this place," I said.

"Will you miss all the exercise?" mum asked.

"Nope."

I looked over at Tracie who seemed lost in a world of her own, presumably reliving that moment at the 1988 Olympics when it all went wrong.

"Do you have to do a lot of exercise to lose weight?" I asked. "Only I really do hate it?"

"Yes, Good question," said mum. "And also - which is best - exercising or dieting to lose weight?"

"Well," she said. "You'll be relieved to hear that there's been a study."

"Hooray!" said mum and I.

She laughed. "I'm not that bad, am I? Forever quoting studies."

"No, not bad - it's good," I said quickly. I'm delighted that you've read all these studies."

"Good, well - this was a big study - done in the UK and featuring more than 300,000 patients. The question they asked was: 'Can weight and inactivity be considered separate risks?' In other words - you can exercise and still be fat and you can be thin and not exercise at all. One does not depend on the other.

"So, the study showed that regular exercise will reduce many of the health risks associated with both being overweight and inactive, but might not directly lead to you losing weight. You have to change your diet to do that.

"This ties in with the other studies that have been done - remember the bus conductor and bus driver study?"

"How could we forget?" I said.

"Well, that was done because drivers were dying earlier, not because they were fatter than conductors. Exercise is important for health and longevity. And you know what else is important?"

"Oooo, do tell," I said.

"The regularity of that exercise. So, if you sit and look at the computer screen for eight hours solid without moving, then go to the gym for an hour, that's not as effective as doing an hour, then some exercise, or having regular exercise breaks through the day. The human body was designed to move."

"So, it would have been ideal if the bus conductors and the drives swapped jobs every hour?" mum said. She can be so wise sometimes.

"Yes - absolutely - that would have saved lives."

"Could it have been stress as well though?" I offer. "I mean - I totally get that exercise is healthy and it's important to build movement into your everyday life, but if I drove a bus all day every day, I'm sure it would be the stress that killed me."

"Back during the bus driver study, stress was not appreciated as a health risk, but you're absolutely right. Things like tight schedules, traffic jams, angry passengers, filthy air and other factors would definitely have been a factor. A life packed with unrelenting stress is far more dangerous than a few extra pounds."

I nodded and smiled, and thanked her for her input, but inside I was thinking 'if I give up work and have no stress in my life, I can eat chocolate all the time.'

WHEN MRS A TURNED UP
UNEXPECTEDLY

It was dinner time. Our last dinner of the trip. It had all gone by so quickly. In many ways, I'd absolutely hated it, but in others, I'd loved it. I'd learned so much, and was kind of looking forward to putting it together in the blog posts next week in the hope that it could help other people.

We walked up to the dining room tables and looked around, working out where to sit. "Hey, come and sit by me," Yvonne called out, tapping the seat next to her and causing me to feel all sorts of anxieties. Did she see mum and me crawling through the hotel bar last night, trying to escape without being seen?

"Come on," I said, dragging mum away from where she had stopped to talk to Simon. I noticed he had his hand on her arm as he spoke to her.

For God's sake, will that man never stop?

"Come on mum, come and sit here."

I treated Simon to an angry scowl and indicated to mum where we would be sitting. I took in the shock on her face as she looked at Yvonne and back to me.

"Had a good day?" she said to Yvonne in a rather forced manner.

"Yes, a lovely day thank you. And you?"

"Yes, it's been great," said Mum.

"How's your eye feeling now."

"Much better, thank you. It looks much worse than it feels."

"I didn't see you both this morning," she said to me. "Did you decide to take it easy?"

"I went with mum to find a doctor," I said. "Then we ended up going on a bit of a mission."

Despite promising myself that I would keep my synchronised swimming story to myself, I couldn't help it.

"Oooo…do tell," said Yvonne. I paused my revelations while chef delivered an unbelievably bland looking bowl of what I assume to be soup, but looked like slosh, then continued once he'd left.

"Well there's been this great mystery going on in our villa," I said. "When I got back after the first night, do you remember I went back early because I haven't been very well?"

"Yes, I remember," said Yvonne. "You fell with an almighty thud and we all thought you died."

"I prefer to think of it as me having delicately fainted, but yes – I collapsed. And when I went back to our villa…"

"I need to stop you there," said mum. Will these people ever stop interrupting my story? "You went back to the wrong villa and climbed into Donald's bed."

"Yes, well – after that, when I got back to my villa."

"Hang on, so – the rumours about you and Donald are true? I assumed they weren't…"

"What rumours? No. No. There is definitely nothing going on between me and Donald. I just went back to the wrong villa, went into what I thought was my room and got into bed. That's all."

"And Donald got in beside you?"

"No. I woke up when he came in, and left."

"That's not strictly true, is it?" said mum. "You did stay there for a little bit, and chat to him when he was in the bed."

"No, look – this is all a distraction. Do you want me to tell you my story about what we got up to this morning or not? It's far more interesting than any half-made-up tale about me accidentally going back to the wrong villa."

"Okay, sorry – carry on," said Yvonne. "We can come back to your love affair with Donald later." She nudged mum and they both giggled at this point but I was determined not to be thrown.

"Well, anyway, when I got back to my room on the first night, the room felt really stuffy, so I opened the patio windows."

Are you sure you weren't just all hot and bothered from your night of passion with Donald?" said Mum.

"No, I was hot because my roommate had forgotten to put the air-conditioning on."

"Oh yes," said Mum. "I just thought it was such a waste of money to leave the air-conditioning on when we were there. It hadn't occurred to me that it would be like a sauna when we got back."

I glared at mum, but Yvonne put her arm round her conspiratorially and said, "It's an easy mistake to make. Almost easy as accidentally getting into a man's bed."

"Can I carry on with my story now?"

"Yes, go on dear," said Mum.

"When I stepped outside and wandered towards the pool, I could see there was a woman in there doing synchronised swimming."

"What?" said Yvonne. "That's so weird... How could there have been someone in there doing synchronised swimming?"

"I know! It was very odd. I sat on the edge of the sun lounger for a while, just watching, but when I moved closer to the pool, the woman saw me and swam like a mad thing towards the edge, climbed out and ran away into the trees. I stood up, and went to go after her, but she'd disappeared."

"I thought she'd gone completely mad," said mum. "You know these people who collapse and have a bang on the head and then are never quite the same afterwards? We thought that's what had happened to Mary."

"I knew I was right though," I said. "I watched for five or 10 minutes, and she was really good, I definitely hadn't imagined it."

"Okay, so what happened next?" said Yvonne. I'd obviously piqued her interest.

"The same thing happened the next night, and again I was on my own, and when I told mum she thought I must have lost my mind. But then last night mum was with me and we saw the swimmer again in the pool."

"Oh, and she was wonderful," said mum. "Very beautiful, gliding through the water in the moonlight she looked like someone in the Olympics you know with a sudden spring up out of the water with a mad smile? She was doing all of that."

I explained to Yvonne how we walked over to stand near the pool, to get a better look, and the swimmer saw us and fled again, but this time she left behind her swimming cap and inside were these initials..."

Just as I was about to continue with the story, Yvonne's phone buzzed into action, and she looked down at it where there was a text message.

"I'm so sorry, I'm dying to hear the end of your story, but I have to go, can you tell me all about it at breakfast?"

"Sure," I said, glancing at mum who immediately looked at me. "I'll tell you the end of the story in the morning."

"Okay, I'll see you then. Sorry to run out. Have a lovely evening."

With that, she was gone, speeding out of the villa.

I looked at mum. "Well I think we know where she's going," I said. "She must be going to meet him again. You can't tell me that she suddenly, desperately, felt the urge to have a sauna."

"No, you're right dear," said Mum.

"And, by the way - stop mentioning the whole Donald thing. Nothing happened it was a simple mistake."

"OK," said mum. "And actually synchronised swimming woman didn't even come that first night, did she? It was the night afterwards. You only saw her once before I was with you. You're losing your mind. I'm the old one – you're supposed to be the one with a good memory."

As we sat there looking at one another, we saw Staff A leave. He walked nonchalantly out of the room then ran up the stone steps, turning a sharp left at the top.

"Do you think we should follow them again?" I said to mum. "It worked out so well last time."

"Ha, ha," she said. "Which bit of it did you think worked out well then?"

"You know the one thing that confuses me about their affair - why aren't they sneaking back to his room? Why would they run off like that, then just sit in a bar? It seems crazy."

"Yes, that is odd," said mum. "Unless they have a room in the hotel?"

"Oh yes. That's probably what they're up to. Oh, go on. Let's follow them again. It's such fun," I said. "I get a real thrill from it. Today was hysterical - finding Tracie. I can't believe how that happened."

As mum and I sat there chatting, a middle-aged woman appeared in the doorway with an overnight bag, looking around, confused. She was wasn't anyone I recognised from the course, and she didn't look as if she worked at the villa.

"Hello, are you looking for Abi?" I said.

As I spoke, Abi came out of the kitchen and saw the lady.

"Anne!" she cried. "How lovely to see you, I didn't realise you were coming."

The two women hugged warmly and she put down her bag.

"I wasn't planning to, but I thought I'd surprise him. I thought we could spend the evening together."

"Oh, he will be delighted," said Abi. "I'm not sure where he is actually. Let me see if I can find out."

Abi disappeared, and Anne sat herself down at a table near the door.

"How are you feeling then, now we're at the end of the week. We managed to get through it all, with only a few minor disasters," said mum.

"OK. I actually quite enjoyed it in the end. Except for boxing. Dad's going to have a fit when he sees your eye," I said.

"I know. I have warned him what to expect when he picks us up at the airport."

As we talked, Abi came up to us. "Have you seen Staff A?" she asked.

I looked at mum and we both looked back at her.

"I think he might have gone out for a walk," I said eventually.

Neither of us wanted to lie, but neither of us wanted to say where he was either, in case he wasn't supposed to be there.

Anne stood up from the table, and walked over to join us.

"This is Anne, Staff A's wife," she said.

"Ohhhh!" I said.

"Nice to meet you," mum said, in a much more controlled fashion.

Then Simon walked over. "I think he's gone down to the hotel bar by the seafront," he said. "He pops down there most evenings to catch up with friends."

"Are you sure?" I said. "He's probably not. He's probably just in his room."

"No – he's not in his room – I just checked," said Abi. "I needed to ask him something, but he's not there. Let me get my jacket, and we'll walk down to the seafront and take a look," Abi said to Anne. "I'll just be a minute."

"You could phone the bar," I suggested. "No need to go down there."

"No – we'll walk. It's a lovely evening."

Abi went to get her jacket and I looked at mum.

"Shall we go," I said to her, while grabbing my hoodie, nodding at Anne, and speed walking towards the door.

"Where are we going?" said mum, running to catch up with me.

"We have to warn them," I said. "We can't let his wife walk in on them."

"OK, you go ahead. My laces are undone. I'll do them up and be right behind you."

I ran ahead of mum, and bolted down the street. Somehow, I was given speed and strength by the mission to get to the amorous lovers before Anne. I ran like the wind - across the gravelly paths and over the grass verges, then down towards the seafront bar on a mission to save a man's marriage.

THE TRUTH ABOUT YVONNE

I burst into the bar and there sat Staff A and Yvonne, holding hands over the table, and looking at one another adoringly.

"Hey," I screamed as I fell towards their table, barely able to talk after all that running. "Move apart, move apart," I shouted. "She'll be here any minute."

Everyone in the bar looked up as I confronted them. I was red in the face and sweating profusely as I started physically manhandling Staff A in an effort to move him away from Yvonne.

"Mary what on earth's the matter?" I couldn't move him. I was panting like a wild animal on a hunt.

"Your wife. She's here," I spluttered, motioning between Staff and Yvonne. I noticed they hadn't stopped holding hands so I leaped in and yanked their hands apart. "For the love of God - do I have to do everything?" I asked, as I saw mum and Mrs A coming into the bar.

"Your wife," I said dramatically, sweeping my hand back to indicate her arrival, before I whispered to Yvonne. "You better run. Quick. It's his wife."

"Hi Anne," said Yvonne, getting up and hugging the woman. "Have you met Mary?" she said.

"Very briefly," said Anne, nodding in my direction.

"Is everything OK?" said a man from the table next to us. I looked up to tell him that everything was fine, when he recognised me. "It's you," he said. "The woman from last night - the one who flashed her bottom at everyone in the sauna and crawled out of the bar on her hands and knees. I'm amazed you have the cheek to show your face in here again."

"What?" said Staff A.

"Oh, it's nothing, nothing at all. Mistaken identity," I said.

The man saw mum standing there and gasped. "My goodness - what happened to your eye?"

"Oh that? That's nothing," said mum. "Mary punched me in the face, but it's much better now."

"Punched you in the face? What sort of animal are you?" he asked me.

"Look, it's fine," said Staff A, standing up and putting his hand out to show the man he wanted him to back off. "I can deal with this."

"You need to run, Quickly," I whispered to Yvonne. "Go now. Save yourself."

The man went back to his table, and Staff A pulled over a couple of chairs

"Take a seat," he said. "Let me get you a drink."

"Oooo. A drink? What - a proper drink?"

"Yes, I'll get you a proper drink. What do you want?"

I ordered a large glass of wine and sat back in anticipation. Mum said she'd have a cup of tea. Yvonne got up and walked to the bar with Staff A while mum, Mrs A and I sat there in horrible, painful silence.

"OK, so what's this all about? Why have you come charging down here and attempted to pull me out of my seat? And what's all this about you flashing everyone in the sauna?" asked Staff A, handing me my drink.

I decide not to address the sauna incident. "To be honest, I thought you and Yvonne were having an affair and when your wife arrived in camp, I thought I ought to come down here before her to warn you. Although, I'm guessing that's not what's going on here, is it?"

Staff A exploded into rip-roaring laughter, and put his arm around me in a friendly fashion. "Oh Mary, you are funny. Yvonne's half my age and I've been happily married for 30 years. My God, this woman has stuck with me through thick and thin, I'm not about to mess her around now."

He and Anne held hands and looked at one another.

"But you've been secretly meeting every night, and you said you didn't know Yvonne when you picked her up at the airport, so I knew you weren't friends...I suppose I just assumed..."

"I didn't say that I didn't know her - I said that I'd never met her before. Look, even though I've never met her, I feel like I know her so well because her dad talked about her all the time."

He trailed off at this point, and looked at Yvonne. "Do you mind if I tell them," he said.

"No, that's fine," said Yvonne. "I don't mind at all."

"OK, well I've been in jail for the past six months. I was locked up after an incident in Afghanistan. I was accused of mistreatment of prisoners...something I never did. It was a horrible time. I was accused of things that no one wants to be accused of."

"Waterboarding?" I asked, remembering Staff B's reaction when I had used the word in jest. "Was it something to do with that?"

"I'm not going into any details, Mary. If you read that in the press then I would ignore anything else that you read in the press about me because I was cleared of everything."

"No - I didn't read anything in the press," I said. "Honestly."

"OK, well the facts are that I was found guilty and locked up, but then evidence emerged which proved that I didn't do it, indeed couldn't have done it. That's all I'm saying. I was freed three weeks ago and didn't go back into the army.

"While I was in prison, there was a guy there who saved my life. He kept me strong, and urged me to keep up the appeal. He was Yvonne's dad. I said that when I came out, I would meet up with her and check she was OK. Then I got this job, and it seemed like the perfect job for me. But I wanted to see Yvonne, so I thought the best thing would be to get Yvonne to come out here. We've been meeting so I can tell her all about her dad in prison."

"Oh," I said. "Gosh, I'm really sorry. I didn't know - I was just trying to help, you know. I didn't want Anne to walk in on you. I just...sorry..."

"It's fine," said Yvonne. "I would have told you all about it if you'd asked."

"Oh," I said, turning to mum. "I never thought about asking. Did you?"

Mum shook her head and finished her tea.

"Shall we go back," I said. "Leave these good people to talk."

"Yes," said mum. "I think that's probably for the best. We've done enough interfering for one day. We need to pack, we have an early flight in the morning."

"OK, see you both before you leave," said Staff A.

"You won't be up that early, will you?" said mum. "We have to leave at 7.30am to get our flight."

"Yes - I'll be up. I'm weighing you first thing, remember. We'll see how much weight you've lost."

"Oh yes - how exciting," said mum. "I'm dying to find out."

"Yeah," I said, really regretting the sneaky coke, crisps and jelly babies and Mars bars (OK - I didn't mention the Mars bars and jelly babies but I knew you'd judge me harshly if I did).

FINAL RESULTS

I stood before the scales like an Olympian about to step up to the start line in the Olympic 100m final. The only difference was that this athlete knew she'd been cheating...sneakily eating and drinking through the week when people weren't watching: coke, crisps, Mars bars and jelly babies. I know, I know - it's terrible, and I'd only cheated myself, but I couldn't have survived on the rations they gave us. Honestly, I'd be dead now. Dead. And the staffs would be up for murder. Would they want that on their consciences? No, they wouldn't. Their lives would be ruined by it. I was doing them a favour by eating; saving them from misery and guilt.

In any case I knew I had eaten far less than I usually would, and exercised a tonne more but still - I couldn't possibly have lost more than a few pounds.

I'd sat there as others in the group had lost up to 6lbs. I knew I'd be looking at 2lbs at the most. I was hit by a sudden rush of disappointment in myself, and anger that I hadn't done this properly...just for four days, to see how much weight I could lose. But then there was the whole 'I might die' thing. Maybe this was better.

"On you pop then," said Staff A, like this was some sort of fun adventure I was engaging in.

I stepped onto the scales and watched the numbers whizz up...17 stone, 18 stone, 19 stone...then it slowed down. It stopped just before 20 stone. "You're 19 stone 9lbs," said Staff. I looked at him as if he'd taken leave of his senses.

"That's insane," I said.

"It's pretty good going, Mary. You've lost 9lbs. You're our biggest loser. Well done! Your mum lost 5lbs and you've lost nine, that's a whole stone between you."

There was a ripple of applause behind me and a small shriek of excitement from mum and they presented me with a floral headdress bearing the words 'biggest loser'.

"Thank you," I said. "This has been the most glorious and interesting trip ever."

I turned to Staff A and gave him a big hug and said something I never thought I'd say: "Thank you for pushing me and believing in me."

"Any time," he said.

Mum and I hugged everyone before leaving, then Staff B came out to our cab with us, carrying our bags.

"You're a superstar," I said, hugging him tightly. "Thanks for your support."

"It's been a pleasure," I said. "We're all really looking forward to reading your blog."

"Ha, ha," I said. "Then you'll know exactly what I got up to."

"Indeed," said Staff B, closing the door for us and giving a mock salute as the car drove off.

"When does your blog go up?" asked mum.

"In two days' time," I said. "When I'm safely out of the country."

"What are you going to write in it?"

"I'm going to write about everything," I said. "Every last detail, but mainly I'm going to say how brilliant it was, and how much I learned. It was brilliant, wasn't it?"

"It was fantastic," said mum, giving me a gentle hug. "Thank you for taking me."

"It's a pleasure. I'm so glad you came. I'm never eating carrots again. Not ever."

"Nor me," said mum. "Nor me."

Ends

MORE BERNICE BLOOM?

I hope you enjoyed the books!

IF YOU WANT to learn more about Bernice Bloom (and if you want a free book!), go to: www.bernicebloom.com. And if you enjoyed the book and could leave me a review, that would be brilliant! x

THERE ARE loads more books in the Adorable Fat Girl series & lots more being released all the time.

Books in the series that are OUT NOW:
BOOK ONE: Diary of an Adorable Fat Girl
Mary Brown is funny, gorgeous and bonkers. She's also about six stone overweight. When she realises she can't cross her legs, has trouble bending over to tie her shoelaces without wheezing like an elderly chain-smoker, and discovers that even her hands and feet look fat, it's time to take action. But what action? She's tried every diet under the sun.

This is the story of what happens when Mary joins 'Fat Club' where she meets a cast of funny characters and one particular man who catches her eye.

BOOK TWO: Adventures of an Adorable Fat Girl

Mary can't get into any of the dresses in Zara (she tries and fails. It's messy!). Still, what does she care? She's got a lovely new boyfriend whose thighs are bigger than her's (yes!!!) and all is looking well...except when she accidentally gets herself into several thousand pounds worth of trouble at the silent auction, has to eat her lunch under the table in the pub because Ted's workmates have spotted them, and suffers the indignity of having a young man's testicles dangled into her face on a party boat to Amsterdam. Oh, and then there are all the issues with the hash-cakes and the sex museum. Besides all those things - everything's fine...just fine!

BOOK THREE: Crazy Life of an Adorable Fat Girl

The second course of 'Fat Club' starts and Mary reunites with the cast of funny characters who graced book one. But this time there's a new Fat Club member...a glamorous blonde who Mary takes against.

We also see Mary facing troubles in her relationship with the wonderful Ted, and we discover why she has been suffering from an eating disorder for most of her life. What traumatic incident in Mary's past has caused her all these problems?

The story is tender and warm, but also laugh-out-loud funny. It will resonate with anyone who has dieted, tried to keep up with any sort of exercise programme or spent 10 minutes in a changing room trying to extricate herself from a way too-small garment that she ambitiously tried on and is now completely stuck in.

BOOK FOUR: FIRST THREE BOOKS COMBINED

This is the first three Fat Girl books altogether in one fantastic, funny package

BOOK FIVE: Christmas with Adorable Fat Girl

It's the Adorable Fat Girl's favourite time of year and she embraces it with the sort of thrill and excitement normally reserved for toddlers seeing jelly tots. Our funny, gorgeous and bonkers heroine finds herself dancing from party to party, covered in tinsel, decorating the

Beckhams' Christmas tree, dressing up as Father Christmas, declaring live on This Morning that she's a drug addict and enjoying two Christmas lunches in quick succession. She's the party queen as she stumbles wildly from disaster to disaster. A funny little treasure to see you smiling through the festive period.

BOOK SIX: Adorable Fat Girl shares her Weight Loss Tips

as well as having a crazy amount of fun at Fat Club, Mary also loses weight...a massive 40lbs!! How does she do it? Here in this mini book - for the first time - she describes the rules that helped her. Also included are the stories of readers who have written in to share their weight loss stories. This is a kind approach to weight loss. It's about learning to love yourself as you shift the pounds. It worked for Mary Brown and everyone at Fat Club (even Ted who can't go a day without a bag of chips and thinks a pint isn't a pint without a bag of pork scratchings). I hope it works for you, and I hope you enjoy it.

BOOK SEVEN: Adorable Fat Girl on Safari

Mary Brown, our fabulous, full-figured heroine, is off on safari with an old school friend. What could possibly go wrong? Lots of things, it turns out. Mary starts off on the wrong foot by turning up dressed in a ribbon bedecked bonnet, having channeled Meryl Streep from Out of Africa. She falls in lust with a khaki-clad ranger half her age and ends up stuck in a tree wearing nothing but her knickers, while sandwiched between two inquisitive baboons. It's never dull...

BOOK EIGHT: Cruise with an Adorable Fat Girl

Mary is off on a cruise. It's the trip of a lifetime...featuring eat-all-you-can buffets and a trek through Europe with a 96-year-old widower called Frank and a flamboyant Spanish dancer called Juan Pedro. Then there's the desperately handsome captain, the appearance of an ex-boyfriend on the ship, the time she's mistaken for a Hollywood film star in Lisbon and tonnes of clothes shopping all over Europe.

BOOK NINE: Adorable Fat Girl Takes up Yoga

The Adorable Fat Girl needs to do something to get fit. What about yoga? I mean - really - how hard can that be? A bit of chanting, some toe touching and a new leotard. Easy! She signs up for a weekend retreat, packs up assorted snacks and heads for the countryside to get in touch with her chi and her third eye. And that's when it all goes wrong. Featuring frantic chickens, an unexpected mud bath, men in loose-fitting shorts and no pants, calamitous headstands, a new bizarre friendship with a yoga guru and a quick hospital trip.

BOOK TEN FIRST THREE HOLIDAY BOOKS COMBINED

This is a combination book containing three of the books in my holiday series: Adorable Fat Girl on Safari, Cruise with an Adorable Fat Girl and Adorable Fat Girl takes up Yoga.

BOOK ELEVEN: Adorable Fat Girl and the Mysterious Invitation

Mary Brown receives an invitation to a funeral. The only problem is: she has absolutely no idea who the guy who's died is. She's told that the deceased invited her on his deathbed, and he's very keen for her to attend, so she heads off to a dilapidated old farm house in a remote part of Wales. When she gets there, she discovers that only five other people have been invited to the funeral. None of them knows who he is either.

NO ONE GOING TO THIS FUNERAL HAS EVER HEARD OF THE DECEASED.

Then they are told that they have 20 hours to work out why they have been invited in order to inherit a million pounds.

Who is this guy and why are they there? And what of the ghostly goings on in the ancient old building?

BOOK TWELVE Adorable Fat Girl goes to weight loss camp

Mary Brown heads to Portugal for a weight loss camp and discovers it's nothing like she expected. "I thought it would be Slimming World in the sunshine, but this is bloody torture," she says, after boxing, running, sand training (sand training?), more running, more star jumps and eating nothing but carrots. Mary wants to hide from the instructors and cheat the system. The trouble is, her mum is with her, and won't leave her alone for a second. Then there's the angry instructor with the deep, dark secret about why he left the army; and the mysterious woman who sneaks into their pool and does synchronised swimming every night. Who the hell is she? Why's she in their pool? And what about Yvonne - the slim, attractive lady who disappears every night after dinner. Where's she going? And what unearthly difficulties will Mary get herself into when she decides to follow her to find out...

BOOK THIRTEEN: The first two weight loss books:
This is Weight loss tips and Weight loss camp together

BOOK FOURTEEN: Mary Brown is single and ready to mingle. Her lovely relationship with Ted is over and she feels lonely and fed up. There's only one thing for it – she decides to launch herself onto the dating scene. But internet dating is not always a warm and cuddly place for a larger lady. Featuring nine dates in nine days, followed by a huge, entirely inadvisable party at the end. It's internet dating like you've never known it before. The question is - will Mary find love?

All available on Amazon now

Is romance your thing?

If it is, see my new romantic novels under the pen name, Rosie Taylor-Kennedy - I've written a series of books about four sisters who live together in Sunshine Cottage in a beautiful village called 'Cove Bay.' It's like Little Women for the modern reader! See Amazon for more details:

And there are lots more books on the way, including Mary's Road Trip to USA with Ted and another mystery for Mary to solve, called Adorable Fat Girl and the Mysterious Pregnancy, and Confessions of an Adorable Fat Girl

Then there's the relaunch of a very funny series of books about Wags...

See the website www.bernicebloom.com

. . .

AND make sure you come and join the Facebook group, full of great, fun women:

Search Bernice Bloom books on Facebook

https://www.facebook.com/BerniceBloombooks

** Thank you so much for all your support **